# Easy Calorie & Protein Counter

### By Helena Schaar

A superior calorie & nutrient counter. Alphabetical listings for fast and easy calorie, carbohydrate, fat, fiber, and protein counts. All your favorite foods, fast food restaurants, beverages, and alcohol. Contains about 3,500 listings. Slim sized to fit in a purse or briefcase, or download the ebook to your favorite device.

"EASY Lifetime Diet & Exercise Guide" included inside in this book. The food counter and fitness guide provides the power for a lifetime of total success controlling your weight!

Written based on extensive research and input from nutritionists and fitness trainers. Includes important tips from people in their 20's, 30's, 40's, and 50's who have defied the odds and remained lean, toned, athletic, and healthy their entire lives. Read all of their secrets here. Read about what really works for lifetime weight control!

# Easy Calorie, Carb, Fat, Fiber, & Protein Counter

## TABLE OF CONTENTS

- **Introduction**

- **Abbreviation Key**

- **Calorie, Carb, Fat, Fiber, & Protein Counters**
  Beverages
  Foods
  Fast Food Restaurants

- **EASY Lifetime Diet & Exercise Guide**
  Healthy Diet Basics
  All About Calories & Weight
  Calorie Expenditure & Exercise
  Weight Loss Secrets
  Ideal Body Weight Chart

# Introduction

Welcome to the **Easy Calorie, Carb, Fat, Fiber, & Protein Counter**. Here is the power to control your weight forever. This is a guide to safe, simple, effective methods of managing weight, while promoting optimal health.

Nutrition experts agree, calories count first in weight management. This book is designed to help count calories accurately, quickly, and easily. Alphabetical listings make locating foods simple. To improve clarity and speed in locating food choices, the tables in this book are divided into 3 sections:

> **Beverages**
> **Foods**
> **Fast Food Restaurants**

Counting calories is a time-honored method for weight management. Nutrition experts agree that calories count first when trying to manage your weight. Other factors can then be addressed, including activity level, and how to balance the intake of carbohydrates, protein, fat, sodium, and other nutrients.

This book is designed to help make counting calories and other nutrients fast and easy. Precise and accurate alphabetical listings provide for quick calorie counts. Whether a pro or a novice at counting calories and nutrients, this book contains all the information needed. In the tables are all the foods people love to eat in the most common serving sizes. This includes the most popular foods, the most common foods, favorite fast food restaurants, brand names, beverages, and alcoholic beverages. There are about 3,500 listings in all.

To use this food counter, simply locate the choice of food or beverage in one of the three alphabetical sections:

**Beverages**
**Foods**
**Fast Food Restaurants**

Managing weight is so much easier with the right tools, including a good calorie/nutrient counter, and a simple exercise plan. This food counter includes the EASY Lifetime Diet & Exercise Guide. Here, find all of the essential tools to manage weight, and shed those unwanted pounds and inches forever. This book is the power base for building a lifetime of good health, and the joy of achieving ideal body weight. The EASY Lifetime Diet & Exercise Guide also gives all the essential information needed to understand calories, healthy dieting, and exercise.

The formulas are included to calculate daily caloric requirements for achieving and maintaining ideal weight. Calorie expenditure is also covered, including how to burn calories faster. Also information about lifestyle activity factors, and how to increase activity levels to burn calories faster. Tips about safe and easy exercise, and plenty of diet tips and secrets. Calorie counting along with a simple exercise routine results in healthy weight management, with long-lasting results.

For the best results, read over the book, and especially, look at favorite foods, to get an idea of which foods are high in calories and which foods are low in calories. That will help make smart food choices every time you eat.

# NOTES:

All listings are medium size or average portion size, unless specifically noted.

"Cooked" means the food is cooked without added fats, sauces, or sugars. This includes boiling, steaming, and heating in a microwave oven.

"Baked" and "Broiled" describe the normal methods of baking and broiling, using nonstick cooking spray, or minimal cooking oil. No other fats, sauces, or sugars added.

References for compiling this book include the United States Department of Agriculture (USDA) nutritional database, food manufacturers nutrient labels, and restaurants printed nutritional data. References for the diet and exercise data include the USDA database, WebMD, recommendations from nutrition and exercise experts, and interviews with successful dieters age 20 to 60 years old.

The data is accurate at the time publication, however, food manufacturers may change their ingredients at any time without notice.

# Abbreviation key

| | |
|---|---|
| appx | approximately |
| as prep | prepared as instructed on package; the usual method |
| avg | average size |
| bev | beverage |
| cal | calorie |
| carb | carbohydrate |
| dia | diameter |
| fl oz | fluid ounce |
| g | gram(s) |
| " | inch(es) |
| Lb | pound |
| Lg | large |
| mcg | microgram(s) |
| med | medium |
| misc | miscellaneous |
| mg | milligram(s) |
| ml | milliliter(s) |
| oz | ounce |
| pc | piece |
| pkg | package |
| pkt | packet |
| prep | prepared |
| sm | small |
| svg | serving |
| sq | square |
| Tbsp | tablespoon |
| Tr | trace- less than 1 g or mg |
| tsp | teaspoon |
| w/ | with |
| w/o | without |

## Metric Conversion Factors:

| Volume | Multiply By | To Find Equivalent |
|---|---|---|
| Teaspoons | 4.93 | Milliliters |
| Tablespoons | 14.79 | Milliliters |
| Fluid ounces | 29.57 | Milliliters |
| Cups | 0.24 | Liters |
| Gallons | 3.79 | Liters |

| Weight | Multiply By | To Find Equivalent |
|---|---|---|
| Ounces | 28.35 | Grams |
| Pounds | 0.45 | Kilograms |

## Approximate Measure Equivalents:

Volume

1 Teaspoon = ...................................5 ml
1 Tablespoon =.....3 Teaspoons =............15 ml
2 Tablespoons =....1 fl oz = .................30 ml
4 Tablespoons =....¼ Cup = ...2 fl oz = .....59 ml
16 Tablespoons =...1 Cup = ...8 fl oz =.....237 ml
1 Cup =..........½ Pint =.......8 fl oz = ..... 237 ml
2 Cups =.........1 Pint =.......16 fl oz = .....474 ml
2 Pints = .........1 Quart =....32 fl oz = ...  946 ml
1 Gallon = ......4 Quarts =..128 fl oz =   3.79 Liters

Weight

1 Ounce = 28 grams
1 Pound = 454 grams

# BEVERAGES

| BEVERAGE:<br>(See Food and Fast Food<br>Restaurants listed separately) | Serv-ing Size | Cal-ories | Fat (g) | Carb (g) | Fi-ber (g) | Pro-tein (g) |
|---|---|---|---|---|---|---|
| Amaretto, 53 proof | 1.5 fl oz | 175 | Tr | 24 | 0 | Tr |
| Apple Juice | 8 fl oz | 115 | Tr | 29 | Tr | Tr |
| Apple-Cranberry Juice | 8 fl oz | 115 | Tr | 29 | Tr | Tr |
| Apple-Grape Juice | 8 fl oz | 130 | Tr | 31 | Tr | Tr |
| Apple-Raspberry Juice | 8 fl oz | 120 | Tr | 30 | Tr | Tr |
| Apricot Nectar | 8 fl oz | 140 | Tr | 36 | Tr | Tr |
| **BEER** | ... | ... | . | . | . | . |
| Regular Beer | 12 fl oz | 150 | 0 | 13 | 1 | 1 |
| Light Beer | 12 fl oz | 100 | 0 | 6 | 0 | 1 |
| Dark beer | 12 fl oz | 160 | 0 | 14 | Tr | 1 |
| Draft beer, regular | 12 fl oz | 150 | 0 | 13 | Tr | 1 |
| Draft beer, light | 12 fl oz | 100 | 0 | 6 | 0 | 1 |
| Dry beer | 12 fl oz | 130 | 0 | 8 | Tr | 1 |
| Malt beer | 12 fl oz | 160 | 0 | 10 | Tr | 1 |
| Bloody Mary | 5 fl oz | 150 | Tr | 5 | Tr | 1 |
| Bourbon, 80 proof | 1.5 fl oz | 95 | 0 | 0 | 0 | 0 |
| Brandy | ... | ... | . | . | . | . |
| 80 proof | 1.5 fl oz | 95 | 0 | 0 | 0 | 0 |
| Flavored, 60 proof, (Apricot<br>Blackberry, or Cherry) | ...<br>1.5 fl oz | ...<br>180 | Tr. | 24 | 0 | Tr |
| Capri Sun juice drink | 8 fl oz | 122 | Tr | 31 | Tr | Tr |
| Carbonated Beverages- see Soda | ... | ... | . | . | . | . |
| Carrot Juice | 8 fl oz | 95 | Tr | 22 | 2 | 2 |
| Club Soda | 12 fl oz | 0 | 0 | 0 | 0 | 0 |
| Cocoa / Chocolate Beverage, Hot | ... | ... | . | . | . | . |
| Regular, as prep | 6 fl oz | 170 | 7 | 23 | 1 | 7 |
| Diet or sugarfree, as prep | 6 fl oz | 35 | 0 | 5 | Tr | 3 |
| **COFFEE** | ... | ... | . | . | . | . |
| Brewed coffee, regular or decaf | 6 fl oz | 4 | 0 | 1 | 0 | Tr |
| Instant coffee, regular or decaf | 6 fl oz | 4 | 0 | 1 | 0 | Tr |
| Café Amaretto | 6 fl oz | 70 | 2 | 6 | 0 | 7 |
| Café Latte | 6 fl oz | 115 | 6 | 10 | 0 | 6 |
| Café Vienna | 6 fl oz | 70 | 2 | 6 | 0 | 7 |
| Cappuccino | 6 fl oz | 65 | 3 | 6 | 0 | 3 |
| Espresso | 2 fl oz | 5 | Tr | 1 | 0 | Tr |
| French Vanilla Café | 6 fl oz | 70 | 2 | 6 | 0 | 7 |

| BEVERAGE:<br>(See Food and Fast Food<br>Restaurants listed separately) | Serv-<br>ing<br>Size | Cal-<br>ories | Fat<br>(g) | Carb<br>(g) | Fi-<br>ber<br>(g) | Pro-<br>tein<br>(g) |
|---|---|---|---|---|---|---|
| French Vanilla, sugarfree | 6 fl oz | 20 | Tr | 4 | 0 | Tr |
| Hazelnut Belgian Cafe | 6 fl oz | 75 | 2 | 7 | 0 | 7 |
| Swiss Mocha coffee | 6 fl oz | 75 | 1 | 8 | Tr | 9 |
| Swiss Mocha coffee, sugarfree | 6 fl oz | 20 | Tr | 4 | 0 | Tr |
| Viennese Chocolate coffee | 6 fl oz | 75 | 1 | 8 | Tr | 9 |
| Coffee Cream – see Creamer | … | … | . | . | . | . |
| Coffee Liqueur, 53 proof | 1.5 fl oz | 175 | Tr | 24 | 0 | Tr |
| Coke - see Soda | … | … | . | . | . | . |
| Cola - see Soda | … | … | . | . | . | . |
| Cranapple Drink | 8 fl oz | 170 | 0 | 43 | Tr | 0 |
| Cranberry Juice Cocktail | 8 fl oz | 145 | Tr | 36 | Tr | 0 |
| Cranberry-Grape Drink | 8 fl oz | 145 | Tr | 34 | Tr | Tr |
| Creamer | … | … | . | . | . | . |
| Half & Half (cream & milk) | 1 Tbsp | 20 | 2 | 1 | 0 | 1 |
| Half & Half (cream & milk) | 1 cup | 315 | 28 | 10 | 0 | 7 |
| Liquid creamer Coffee-Mate | 1 Tbsp | 20 | 1 | 2 | 0 | Tr |
| Powdered creamer Coffee-Mate | 1 tsp | 10 | Tr | 2 | 0 | Tr |
| Crème de Menthe | 1 fl oz | 125 | 0 | 14 | 0 | 0 |
| Crystal Light, all flavors | 8 fl oz | 5 | 0 | 0 | 0 | 0 |
| Daiquiri, strawberry | 4 fl oz | 225 | Tr | 8 | Tr | Tr |
| Diet Cola | 12 fl oz | 0 | 0 | 0 | 0 | 0 |
| Diet or sugarfree Kool Aid | 8 fl oz | 5 | 0 | 1 | Tr | 0 |
| Diet Soda | 12 fl oz | 0 | 0 | 0 | 0 | 0 |
| Eggnog, plain | 1 cup | 345 | 19 | 34 | 0 | 10 |
| Fruit Drink (5% to 10% juice) | … | … | . | . | . | . |
| All flavors | … | … | . | . | . | . |
| Regular | 8 fl oz | 135 | 0 | 32 | Tr | 0 |
| Sugarfree | 8 fl oz | 5 | 0 | 1 | Tr | 0 |
| Fruit Punch (10% Juice) | … | … | . | . | . | . |
| Regular | 8 fl oz | 130 | 0 | 31 | Tr | 0 |
| Sugarfree | 8 fl oz | 5 | 0 | 1 | Tr | 0 |
| Gatorade | 8 fl oz | 50 | 0 | 14 | 0 | 0 |
| Gin, 80 proof | 1.5 fl oz | 95 | 0 | 0 | 0 | 0 |
| Grape Juice | … | … | . | . | . | . |
| Canned or bottled, sweetened | 8 fl oz | 155 | Tr | 38 | Tr | 1 |
| Frozen concentrate, sweetened, | … | … | . | . | . | . |
| as prep w/ water | 8 fl oz | 130 | Tr | 32 | Tr | Tr |
| Unsweetened grape juice | 8 fl oz | 120 | Tr | 30 | Tr | Tr |
| Grapefruit Juice | … | … | . | . | . | . |
| Fresh, squeezed, unsweetened | 8 fl oz | 95 | Tr | 22 | Tr | 1 |

| BEVERAGE:<br>(See Food and Fast Food Restaurants listed separately) | Serv-ing Size | Cal-ories | Fat (g) | Carb (g) | Fi-ber (g) | Pro-tein (g) |
|---|---|---|---|---|---|---|
| Fresh, squeezed, sugar sweetened | ...<br>8 fl oz | ...<br>115 | .<br>Tr | .<br>28 | .<br>Tr | .<br>1 |
| Fresh, squeezed, w/sugarfree sweetener | ...<br>8 fl oz | ...<br>90 | .<br>Tr | .<br>22 | .<br>Tr | .<br>1 |
| Canned, unsweetened | 8 fl oz | 95 | Tr | 22 | Tr | 1 |
| Canned, sugar sweetened | 8 fl oz | 115 | Tr | 28 | Tr | 1 |
| Frozen concentrate, unsweetened, as prep w/ water | ...<br>8 fl oz | .<br>100 | .<br>Tr | .<br>24 | .<br>Tr | .<br>1 |
| Half & Half – see Creamer | ... | ... | . | . | . | . |
| Hawaiian Punch | ... | ... | . | . | . | . |
| Regular | 8 fl oz | 120 | 0 | 30 | Tr | 0 |
| Sugarfree | 8 fl oz | 15 | 0 | 4 | Tr | 0 |
| Hot Cocoa/Chocolate – see | ... | ... | . | . | . | . |
| Cocoa | ... | ... | . | . | . | . |
| Juice – see specific listings | ... | ... | . | . | . | . |
| Kool Aid | ... | ... | . | . | . | . |
| Sugar sweetened | 8 fl oz | 60 | 0 | 16 | Tr | 0 |
| Sugarfree | 8 fl oz | 5 | 0 | 1 | Tr | 0 |
| Unsweetened Packet | 1 pkt | 0 | 0 | 0 | 0 | 0 |
| Lemon Juice | ... | ... | . | . | . | . |
| Fresh, squeezed, unsweetened | 1 Tbsp | 4 | Tr | 1 | Tr | Tr |
| Canned or bottled, unsweetened | 1 Tbsp | 3 | Tr | 1 | Tr | Tr |
| Canned or bottled, unsweetened | 1 cup | 50 | 1 | 16 | 1 | 1 |
| Lemonade | ... | ... | . | . | . | . |
| Sugar Sweetened | 8 fl oz | 100 | 0 | 25 | Tr | 0 |
| Sugarfree | 8 fl oz | 5 | 0 | 1 | Tr | 0 |
| Lime Juice | ... | ... | . | . | . | . |
| Fresh or bottled, unsweetened | 1 Tbsp | 3 | Tr | 1 | Tr | Tr |
| Fresh or bottled, unsweetened | 1 cup | 52 | 1 | 16 | 1 | 1 |
| Limeade | ... | ... | . | . | . | . |
| Sugar sweetened | 8 fl oz | 100 | 0 | 25 | Tr | 0 |
| Sugarfree | 8 fl oz | 5 | 0 | 1 | Tr | 0 |
| Liqueur, 53 proof | ... | ... | . | . | . | . |
| Coffee or Fruit Flavored | 1.5 fl oz | 175 | Tr | 24 | 0 | Tr |
| Mai Tai | 5 fl oz | 280 | Tr | 28 | 1 | 1 |
| Margarita | 5 fl oz | 150 | 0 | 10 | Tr | 0 |
| Martini | 2.5 fl oz | 155 | 0 | 0 | 0 | 0 |
| MILK | ... | ... | . | . | . | . |
| White Milk | ... | ... | . | . | . | . |
| Whole milk, 3.3% fat | 8 fl oz | 150 | 8 | 11 | 0 | 8 |

| BEVERAGE:<br>(See Food and Fast Food<br>Restaurants listed separately) | Serv-<br>ing<br>Size | Cal-<br>ories | Fat<br>(g) | Carb<br>(g) | Fi-<br>ber<br>(g) | Pro-<br>tein<br>(g) |
|---|---|---|---|---|---|---|
| Reduced fat milk, 2% fat | 8 fl oz | 120 | 5 | 12 | 0 | 8 |
| Lowfat milk, 1% fat | 8 fl oz | 102 | 3 | 12 | 0 | 8 |
| Nonfat milk, (Skim milk) | 8 fl oz | 85 | Tr | 12 | 0 | 8 |
| Nonfat instant,as prep w/water | 8 fl oz | 80 | 0 | 12 | 0 | 8 |
| Nonfat instant, | ... | ... | ... | ... | ... | ... |
| dry powder only | 1 cup | 240 | 0 | 36 | 0 | 24 |
| Chocolate Milk | ... | ... | . | . | . | . |
| Whole chocolate milk | 8 fl oz | 210 | 8 | 26 | 2 | 8 |
| Reduced fat chocolate,2% | 8 fl oz | 180 | 5 | 26 | 1 | 8 |
| Lowfat chocolate milk, 1% | 8 fl oz | 160 | 3 | 26 | 1 | 8 |
| Misc Milk Products | ... | ... | . | . | . | . |
| Buttermilk | 1 cup | 100 | 2 | 12 | 0 | 8 |
| Condensed, sweetened | 1 cup | 980 | 27 | 166 | 0 | 24 |
| Evaporated whole milk | 1 cup | 340 | 19 | 25 | 0 | 17 |
| Evaporated skim milk | 1 cup | 200 | 1 | 29 | 0 | 19 |
| Malted milk, chocolate | 1 cup | 225 | 9 | 29 | Tr | 9 |
| Malted milk, natural | 1 cup | 230 | 9 | 28 | 0 | 10 |
| Soy milk | 1 cup | 81 | 5 | 4 | 3 | 7 |
| Milk Shake – see Shake | ... | ... | . | . | . | . |
| Miso | 1 cup | 567 | 17 | 77 | 15 | 32 |
| Nesquik, Chocolate, as prep | 8 fl oz | 210 | 5 | 33 | 1 | 7 |
| Orange Juice | ... | ... | . | . | . | . |
| Fresh, squeezed, unsweetened | 8 fl oz | 112 | Tr | 26 | 1 | 2 |
| Canned or bottled, unsweetened | 8 fl oz | 110 | Tr | 25 | 1 | 2 |
| Frozen concentrate, as prep | 8 fl oz | 112 | Tr | 26 | 1 | 2 |
| Peach Nectar | 8 fl oz | 135 | 0 | 34 | Tr | 1 |
| Pear Nectar | 8 fl oz | 150 | 0 | 39 | Tr | 0 |
| Pepsi – see  Soda | ... | ... | . | . | . | . |
| Pina Colada | 4.5 oz | 260 | 3 | 40 | 1 | 1 |
| Pineapple Grapefruit Juice | 8 fl oz | 120 | Tr | 29 | Tr | 1 |
| Pineapple Juice | 8 fl oz | 140 | Tr | 34 | 1 | 1 |
| Pineapple Orange Juice | 8 fl oz | 125 | 0 | 30 | Tr | 3 |
| Prune Juice | 8 fl oz | 182 | Tr | 45 | 3 | 2 |
| Root Beer | ... | ... | . | . | . | . |
| Regular | 12 fl oz | 170 | 0 | 47 | 0 | 0 |
| Diet or sugarfree | 12 fl oz | 0 | 0 | 0 | 0 | 0 |
| Rum, 80 proof | 1.5 fl oz | 95 | 0 | 0 | 0 | 0 |
| Scotch,  80 proof | 1.5 fl oz | 95 | 0 | 0 | 0 | 0 |
| Screwdriver | 7 fl oz | 160 | Tr | 17 | 1 | Tr |
| Shake | ... | ... | . | . | . | . |

| BEVERAGE: (See Food and Fast Food Restaurants listed separately) | Serving Size | Calories | Fat (g) | Carb (g) | Fiber (g) | Protein (g) |
|---|---|---|---|---|---|---|
| Regular milk shake | ... | ... | . | . | . | . |
| Chocolate | 11 oz | 360 | 8 | 63 | 1 | 9 |
| Peach | 11 oz | 380 | 4 | 75 | 1 | 10 |
| Strawberry | 11 oz | 395 | 4 | 80 | 1 | 11 |
| Vanilla | 11 0z | 350 | 9 | 56 | 0 | 12 |
| Low Carb shake | ... | ... | . | . | . | . |
| Atkins chocolate shake | 11 oz | 170 | 9 | 5 | 3 | 20 |
| Atkins vanilla shake | 11 oz | 170 | 9 | 4 | 2 | 20 |
| **Soda / Cola / Soft Drink** | ... | ... | . | . | . | . |
| (Carbonated Beverages) | ... | ... | . | . | . | . |
| Club Soda | 12 fl oz | 0 | 0 | 0 | 0 | 0 |
| Cherry Cola, regular | 12 fl oz | 155 | 0 | 40 | 0 | 0 |
| Cherry Cola, diet | 12 fl oz | 0 | 0 | 0 | 0 | 0 |
| Coca Cola, Coke regular | 12 fl oz | 140 | 0 | 39 | 0 | 0 |
| Coke, diet | 12 fl oz | 0 | 0 | 0 | 0 | 0 |
| Cola | 12 fl oz | 150 | 0 | 40 | 0 | 0 |
| Diet Cola | 12 fl oz | 0 | 0 | 0 | 0 | 0 |
| Dr Pepper, regular | 12 fl oz | 150 | 0 | 40 | 0 | 0 |
| Dr Pepper, diet | 12 fl oz | 0 | 0 | 0 | 0 | 0 |
| Ginger Ale, regular | 12 fl oz | 125 | 0 | 32 | 0 | 0 |
| Ginger Ale, diet | 12 fl oz | 0 | 0 | 0 | 0 | 0 |
| Grape Soda, regular | 12 fl oz | 155 | 0 | 40 | 0 | 0 |
| Grape Soda, diet | 12 fl oz | 0 | 0 | 0 | 0 | 0 |
| Lemon Lime Soda, regular | 12 fl oz | 145 | 0 | 36 | 0 | 0 |
| Lemon Lime Soda, diet | 12 fl oz | 0 | 0 | 0 | 0 | 0 |
| Mountain Dew, regular | 12 fl oz | 170 | 0 | 46 | 0 | 0 |
| Mountain Dew, diet | 12 fl oz | 0 | 0 | 0 | 0 | 0 |
| Mr. Pibb, regular | 12 fl oz | 146 | 0 | 39 | 0 | 0 |
| Mr. Pibb, diet | 12 fl oz | 0 | 0 | 0 | 0 | 0 |
| Orange Soda, regular | 12 fl oz | 175 | 0 | 45 | 0 | 0 |
| Orange Soda, diet | 12 fl oz | 0 | 0 | 0 | 0 | 0 |
| Pepsi, regular | 12 fl oz | 150 | 0 | 41 | 0 | 0 |
| Pepsi, diet | 12 fl oz | 0 | 0 | 0 | 0 | 0 |
| RC Cola, regular | 12 fl oz | 160 | 0 | 43 | 0 | 0 |
| RC Cola, diet | 12 fl oz | 0 | 0 | 0 | 0 | 0 |
| Root Beer, Regular | 12 fl oz | 170 | 0 | 44 | 0 | 0 |
| Root Beer, Diet | 12 fl oz | 0 | 0 | 0 | 0 | 0 |
| Seven Up, regular | 12 fl oz | 150 | 0 | 39 | 0 | 0 |
| Seven Up, diet | 12 fl oz | 0 | 0 | 0 | 0 | 0 |
| Sprite, regular | 12 fl oz | 150 | 0 | 39 | 0 | 0 |
| Sprite, diet | 12 fl oz | 0 | 0 | 0 | 0 | 0 |

| BEVERAGE:<br>(See Food and Fast Food<br>Restaurants listed separately) | Serving Size | Calories | Fat (g) | Carb (g) | Fiber (g) | Protein (g) |
|---|---|---|---|---|---|---|
| Tab | 12 fl oz | 1 | 0 | 0 | 0 | 0 |
| Soft Drinks – see Soda | ... | ... | . | . | . | . |
| Sport Drink | 12 fl oz | 75 | 0 | 18 | 0 | 0 |
| Sugarfree Beverage | ... | . | . | . | . | . |
| (Also see specific listings) | ... | . | . | . | . | . |
| Sugarfree Soda | 12 fl oz | 0 | 0 | 0 | 0 | 0 |
| Sugarfree Kool Aid | 8 fl oz | 5 | 0 | 1 | Tr | 0 |
| Sunny Delight, Citrus Punch | 8 fl oz | 125 | 0 | 31 | Tr | 0 |
| Tang, regular | 8 fl oz | 115 | 0 | 29 | Tr | 0 |
| Tang, sugarfree | 8 fl oz | 5 | 0 | Tr | Tr | 0 |
| TEA, Hot or Iced | ... | ... | . | . | . | . |
| Regular, unsweetened | 8 fl oz | 2 | 0 | 1 | 0 | 0 |
| Regular, sugar sweetened | 8 fl oz | 90 | 0 | 22 | 0 | 0 |
| Regular, sugarfree sweetener | 8 fl oz | 4 | 0 | 1 | 0 | 0 |
| Chamomile tea, unsweetened | 8 fl oz | 2 | 0 | Tr | 0 | 0 |
| Chamomile tea, sugar<br>sweetened | 8 fl oz | 90 | 0 | 21 | 0 | 0 |
| Misc Types of Tea, Blends, | ... | ... | . | . | . | . |
| Black, Chinese, Orange Pekoe | ... | ... | . | . | . | . |
| Unsweetened | 8 fl oz | 2 | 0 | Tr | 0 | 0 |
| Sugar sweetened | 8 fl oz | 90 | 0 | 22 | 0 | 0 |
| Sugarfree sweetened | 8 fl oz | 4 | 0 | 1 | 0 | 0 |
| Tequila | 1.5 fl oz | 100 | 0 | 0 | 0 | 0 |
| Tequila Sunrise | 5.5 fl oz | 190 | 0 | 15 | 1 | 1 |
| Tomato Juice | 8 fl oz | 41 | Tr | 10 | 1 | 2 |
| V 8 Vegetable Juice, 1 Lg can | 11 fl oz | 70 | 0 | 15 | 2 | 2 |
| Vegetable Juice | 8 fl oz | 46 | Tr | 11 | 2 | 2 |
| Vodka | ... | ... | . | . | . | . |
| 80 proof | 1.5 oz | 95 | 0 | 0 | 0 | 0 |
| 86 proof | 1.5 oz | 105 | 0 | Tr | 0 | 0 |
| 90 proof | 1.5 oz | 110 | 0 | Tr | 0 | 0 |
| Water | 8 fl oz | 0 | 0 | 0 | 0 | 0 |
| Whiskey | ... | ... | . | . | . | . |
| 80 proof | 1.5 oz | 95 | 0 | 0 | 0 | 0 |
| 86 proof | 1.5 oz | 105 | 0 | Tr | 0 | 0 |
| 90 proof | 1.5 oz | 110 | 0 | Tr | 0 | 0 |
| WINE | ... | ... | . | . | . | . |
| Dessert Wine, Dry | 4 fl oz | 150 | 0 | 5 | 0 | Tr |
| Dessert Wine, Sweet | 4 fl oz | 180 | 0 | 14 | 0 | Tr |
| Red Wine (table wine) | 4 fl oz | 85 | 0 | 2 | 0 | Tr |

| BEVERAGE:<br>(See Food and Fast Food Restaurants listed separately) | Serv-ing Size | Cal-ories | Fat (g) | Carb (g) | Fi-ber (g) | Pro-tein (g) |
|---|---|---|---|---|---|---|
| Rosè Wine | 4 fl oz | 85 | 0 | 1 | 0 | Tr |
| White Wine (table wine) | 4 fl oz | 80 | 0 | 1 | 0 | Tr |
| White Zinfandel | 4 fl oz | 85 | 0 | 1 | 0 | Tr |
| Wine Cooler | 5.5 oz | 100 | 0 | 11 | 0 | Tr |
| Wine Spritzer | 5.5 oz | 60 | 0 | 1 | 0 | Tr |

# FOODS

| FOOD:<br>(See Beverages & Fast Food Restaurants listed separately) | Serv-<br>ing<br>Size | Cal-<br>ories | Fat<br>(g) | Carb<br>(g) | Fi-<br>ber<br>(g) | Pro-<br>tein<br>(g) |
|---|---|---|---|---|---|---|
| Accent Seasoning | ¼ tsp | Tr | 0 | 0 | 0 | 0 |
| Alfalfa sprouts, fresh | 1 cup | 10 | Tr | 1 | Tr | 1 |
| Almonds – see Nuts | ... | ... | . | . | . | . |
| Anchovy – see Fish | ... | ... | . | . | . | . |
| Anise Seed | 1 Tbsp | 28 | 1 | 3 | 1 | 1 |
| Apple | ... | ... | . | . | . | . |
|   Fresh, unpeeled, avg 2 ¾" dia | 1 | 80 | Tr | 21 | 4 | Tr |
|   Fresh, peeled, sliced | 1 cup | 65 | Tr | 16 | 2 | Tr |
|   Dried | 5 rings | 80 | Tr | 21 | 3 | Tr |
| Apple Butter | 1 Tbsp | 30 | 0 | 7 | Tr | Tr |
| Apple Pie Filling | 1 Tbsp | 40 | 1 | 8 | 1 | Tr |
| Applesauce | ... | ... | . | . | . | . |
|   Sweetened | ½ cup | 97 | Tr | 25 | 2 | Tr |
|   Unsweetened | ½ cup | 52 | Tr | 14 | 2 | Tr |
| Apricot | ... | ... | . | . | . | . |
|   Fresh, medium size, 1.3 oz | 1 | 17 | Tr | 4 | 1 | Tr |
|   Canned, in heavy syrup | 1 cup | 215 | Tr | 55 | 4 | 1 |
|   Canned, in juice | 1 cup | 115 | Tr | 30 | 4 | 2 |
|   Dried, halves | 8 halves | 80 | Tr | 21 | 3 | 1 |
| Artichoke, Globe or French | ... | ... | . | . | . | . |
|   Fresh, medium size, cooked | 1 | 60 | Tr | 13 | 7 | 4 |
|   Fresh, cooked, drained | 1 cup | 84 | Tr | 19 | 9 | 6 |
|   Jerusalem artichoke, raw, sliced | 1 cup | 114 | Tr | 26 | 2 | 3 |
| Arugula, raw | ½ cup | 3 | 0 | Tr | Tr | Tr |
| Asparagus, cooked | ... | ... | . | . | . | . |
|   Fresh, medium size spears | 4 spears | 14 | Tr | 3 | 1 | 2 |
|   Fresh, chopped pieces | 1 cup | 43 | 1 | 8 | 3 | 5 |
|   Frozen, spears | 4 spears | 17 | Tr | 3 | 1 | 2 |
|   Frozen, chopped pieces | 1 cup | 50 | 1 | 9 | 3 | 5 |
|   Canned, 5" spears | 4 spears | 14 | Tr | 2 | 1 | 2 |
|   Canned, chopped pieces | 1 cup | 46 | 2 | 6 | 4 | 5 |
| Aspartame Sweetener | 1 pkt | 0 | 0 | Tr | 0 | 0 |
| Avocado | ... | ... | . | . | . | . |
|   California, 1/5 of whole | 1 oz | 50 | 5 | 2 | 1 | 1 |
|   Florida, 1/10 of whole | 1 oz | 30 | 3 | 3 | 1 | Tr |
| Bacon – see Pork | ... | ... | . | . | . | . |
| Bacon Bits | 1 Tbsp | 31 | 2 | 2 | 1 | 2 |

| FOOD: (See Beverages & Fast Food Restaurants listed separately) | Serving Size | Calories | Fat (g) | Carb (g) | Fiber (g) | Protein (g) |
|---|---|---|---|---|---|---|
| Bagel, 3 ½" dia | ... | ... | . | . | . | . |
| Plain | 1 | 150 | 1 | 34 | 2 | 4 |
| Cinnamon raisin | 1 | 170 | 1 | 36 | 2 | 5 |
| Egg | 1 | 160 | 1 | 34 | 2 | 5 |
| Multigrain | 1 | 150 | 1 | 33 | 3 | 5 |
| Baking Powder | 1 tsp | 2 | 0 | 1 | Tr | 0 |
| Baking Soda | 1 tsp | 0 | 0 | 0 | 0 | 0 |
| Bamboo Shoots, cooked | 1 cup | 25 | 1 | 4 | 2 | 2 |
| Banana | ... | ... | . | . | . | . |
| Fresh, 7" long | 1 | 110 | 1 | 28 | 3 | 1 |
| Fresh, sliced | 1 cup | 140 | 1 | 35 | 4 | 2 |
| Banana Split | 1 | 510 | 12 | 96 | 4 | 8 |
| Barley | ... | ... | . | . | . | . |
| Pearled, cooked | 1 cup | 195 | 1 | 44 | 6 | 4 |
| Pearled, uncooked | 1 cup | 705 | 2 | 155 | 31 | 20 |
| Basil, dried spice | ½ tsp | 3 | 0 | Tr | Tr | Tr |
| Bean Sprouts (mung), cooked | 1 cup | 30 | Tr | 5 | 2 | 3 |
| **BEANS** | ... | ... | . | . | . | . |
| Plain Beans, cooked w/o fats | ... | ... | . | . | . | . |
| Black beans | ½ cup | 115 | 1 | 21 | 8 | 7 |
| Great Northern beans | ½ cup | 105 | 1 | 19 | 6 | 7 |
| Green beans | ½ cup | 22 | Tr | 5 | 3 | 1 |
| Kidney, Red beans | ½ cup | 112 | 1 | 20 | 7 | 7 |
| Lima, large beans | ½ cup | 100 | 1 | 17 | 8 | 7 |
| Lima, baby lima beans | ½ cup | 95 | 1 | 17 | 10 | 6 |
| Pinto beans | ½ cup | 117 | 1 | 22 | 7 | 7 |
| Soybeans | ½ cup | 135 | 6 | 10 | 5 | 12 |
| Wax beans | ½ cup | 25 | Tr | 5 | 3 | 1 |
| White beans | ½ cup | 150 | 1 | 28 | 6 | 9 |
| Yellow beans | ½ cup | 22 | Tr | 5 | 3 | 1 |
| Misc Bean Dishes, as prep | ... | ... | . | . | . | . |
| Baked beans, | ... | ... | . | . | . | . |
| plain or vegetarian | ½ cup | 118 | 1 | 26 | 6 | 6 |
| Baked beans, BBQ style | ½ cup | 180 | 3 | 32 | 7 | 5 |
| Baked beans w/frankfurters | ½ cup | 185 | 8 | 20 | 9 | 9 |
| Baked beans w/tomato sauce | ½ cup | 125 | 2 | 25 | 6 | 7 |
| Baked beans w/sweet sauce | ½ cup | 140 | 2 | 27 | 7 | 7 |
| Beans w/ pork | ½ cup | 130 | 2 | 24 | 6 | 5 |
| Black beans w/ rice | ½ cup | 150 | 5 | 23 | 5 | 4 |
| Green bean casserole | ½ cup | 140 | 2 | 13 | 5 | 3 |
| Green beans w/almonds | ½ cup | 60 | 2 | 8 | 4 | 3 |

| FOOD: (See Beverages & Fast Food Restaurants listed separately) | Serving Size | Calories | Fat (g) | Carb (g) | Fiber (g) | Protein (g) |
|---|---|---|---|---|---|---|
| Red beans & rice | ½ cup | 130 | 2 | 23 | 6 | 4 |
| Refried beans | ½ cup | 118 | 2 | 20 | 7 | 7 |
| **BEEF** | ... | ... | . | . | . | . |
| (Weights for meat w/o bones, | ... | ... | . | . | . | . |
| as prep: braised, broiled, | ... | ... | . | . | . | . |
| grilled, simmered, or roasted) | ... | ... | . | . | . | . |
| Bottom Round, lean & fat | 3 oz | 235 | 14 | 0 | 0 | 24 |
| lean only | 3 oz | 180 | 7 | 0 | 0 | 27 |
| Brisket | 3 oz | 250 | 17 | 0 | 0 | 23 |
| Chuck Blade, lean & fat | 3 oz | 295 | 22 | 0 | 0 | 23 |
| lean only | 3 oz | 215 | 11 | 0 | 0 | 26 |
| Corned Beef, canned | 3 oz | 215 | 13 | 0 | 0 | 23 |
| Dried Beef, chipped | 1 oz | 45 | 1 | Tr | 0 | 8 |
| Eye of Round, lean & fat | 3 oz | 195 | 11 | 0 | 0 | 23 |
| lean only | 3 oz | 145 | 4 | 0 | 0 | 25 |
| Flank Steak | 3 oz | 225 | 14 | 0 | 0 | 23 |
| Ground Beef / | ... | ... | . | . | . | . |
| Hamburger meat, regular | 3 oz | 250 | 18 | 0 | 0 | 20 |
| lean, 79% | 3 oz | 230 | 16 | 0 | 0 | 21 |
| extra lean, 83% | 3 oz | 220 | 14 | 0 | 0 | 22 |
| Liver of beef, fried | 3 oz | 185 | 7 | 7 | 0 | 23 |
| Pastrami | 2 oz | 90 | 4 | 2 | Tr | 12 |
| Porterhouse Steak | 3.5 oz | 325 | 26 | 0 | 0 | 22 |
| Pot Roast, Chuck | 3.5 oz | 345 | 26 | 0 | 0 | 27 |
| Prime Ribs | 3.5 oz | 400 | 34 | 0 | 0 | 23 |
| Rib Roast, lean & fat | 3 oz | 305 | 25 | 0 | 0 | 19 |
| lean only | 3 oz | 195 | 11 | 0 | 0 | 23 |
| Roast Beef | 3.5 oz | 290 | 20 | 0 | 0 | 25 |
| Short Ribs | 3.5 oz | 470 | 42 | 0 | 0 | 22 |
| Sirloin Steak, lean & fat | 3 oz | 220 | 13 | 0 | 0 | 24 |
| lean only | 3 oz | 165 | 6 | 0 | 0 | 26 |
| T-bone Steak, lean & fat | 3.5 oz | 310 | 23 | 0 | 0 | 23 |
| lean only | 3.5 oz | 250 | 16 | 0 | 0 | 25 |
| Tenderloin Steak/ Top Loin | 3.5 oz | 305 | 22 | 0 | 0 | 25 |
| Top Round | 3.5 oz | 215 | 9 | 0 | 0 | 32 |
| (Other Beef Products, see: | ... | ... | . | . | . | . |
| Bologna, Hot Dog, Salami, | ... | ... | . | . | . | . |
| Sausage & specific entrées) | ... | ... | . | . | . | . |
| Beef & Macaroni | ... | ... | . | . | . | . |
| Healthy Choice, frozen | 1 pkg | 210 | 2 | 33 | 5 | 14 |
| Beef Burgundy, Le Menu entrée | 1 meal | 315 | 19 | 12 | 1 | 25 |

| FOOD: (See Beverages & Fast Food Restaurants listed separately) | Serv-ing Size | Cal-ories | Fat (g) | Carb (g) | Fi-ber (g) | Pro-tein (g) |
|---|---|---|---|---|---|---|
| Beef Jerky, ¾ oz | 1 | 80 | 5 | 2 | Tr | 7 |
| Beef Meals – see Hamburger Helper for ground beef meals | ... ... | ... ... | . . | . . | . . | . . |
| Beef Oriental, Lean Cuisine | 1 meal | 270 | 8 | 30 | 3 | 20 |
| Beef Patties, Banquet entrée | 1 meal | 180 | 14 | 7 | Tr | 8 |
| Beef Peppercorn, Lean Cuisine | 1 meal | 260 | 7 | 32 | 1 | 16 |
| Beef Portabello, Lean Cuisine | 1 meal | 220 | 7 | 24 | 1 | 14 |
| Beef Romanoff | 1 cup | 290 | 11 | 28 | 2 | 20 |
| Beef Stew w/ Vegetables | 1 cup | 215 | 12 | 16 | 4 | 11 |
| Beef Stroganoff, Stouffers entrée | 1 meal | 390 | 20 | 30 | 1 | 23 |
| Beef Teriyaki w/ vegetables | 1 cup | 250 | 10 | 22 | 3 | 18 |
| Beef Tips, Healthy Choice entrée | 1 meal | 260 | 6 | 32 | 1 | 20 |
| Beef w/ Broccoli, Hunan style | 1 cup | 250 | 8 | 30 | 3 | 18 |
| Beef w/Vegetables, Szechuan | 1 cup | 270 | 8 | 30 | 3 | 20 |
| Beet Greens, chopped, cooked | ½ cup | 20 | Tr | 4 | 2 | 2 |
| Beets | ... | ... | . | . | . | . |
| Fresh, cooked, slices | ½ cup | 38 | Tr | 8 | 2 | 2 |
| Fresh, cooked, whole, 2" dia | 1 whole | 22 | Tr | 5 | 1 | 1 |
| Canned, drained, slices | ½ cup | 27 | Tr | 6 | 1 | 1 |
| Canned, drained, whole beet | 1 whole | 12 | Tr | 2 | Tr | 1 |
| Biscuit,  plain or buttermilk | ... | ... | . | . | . | . |
| Prep from recipe, 2 ½" dia | 1 | 210 | 10 | 27 | 1 | 4 |
| Prep from recipe, 4" dia | 1 | 360 | 16 | 45 | 2 | 7 |
| Refrigerated dough, baked | ... | ... | . | . | . | . |
| regular 2 ½"  dia | 1 | 95 | 4 | 13 | Tr | 2 |
| reduced fat, 2 ¼" dia | 1 | 65 | 1 | 12 | Tr | 2 |
| Biscuit w/ Bacon | 1 | 360 | 4 | 27 | 1 | 9 |
| Biscuit w/ Egg & Sausage | 1 | 540 | 37 | 32 | 1 | 19 |
| Biscuit w/ Ham | 1 | 330 | 20 | 28 | 1 | 12 |
| Biscuit w/ Sausage | 1 | 460 | 33 | 28 | 1 | 12 |
| Blackberries | ... | ... | . | . | . | . |
| Fresh | 1 cup | 75 | 1 | 18 | 8 | 1 |
| Frozen, no sugar added, thawed | 1 cup | 80 | 1 | 19 | 8 | 1 |
| Blueberries | ... | ... | . | . | . | . |
| Fresh | 1 cup | 80 | 1 | 20 | 4 | 1 |
| Frozen, sugar sweetened, thawed | 1 cup | 185 | Tr | 50 | 5 | 1 |
| Bologna   (thin 1/8" slices) | ... | ... | . | . | . | . |
| Beef or Pork, regular | 2 slices | 180 | 16 | 2 | 0 | 7 |
| Beef or Pork, lowfat | 2 slices | 110 | 9 | 2 | 0 | 6 |
| Beef or Pork, fat free | 2 slices | 60 | 1 | 3 | 0 | 8 |

| FOOD:<br>(See Beverages & Fast Food Restaurants listed separately) | Serv-ing Size | Cal-ories | Fat (g) | Carb (g) | Fi-ber (g) | Pro-tein (g) |
|---|---|---|---|---|---|---|
| Chicken or Turkey , regular | 2 slices | 160 | 14 | 2 | 0 | 7 |
| Chicken or Turkey, lowfat | 2 slices | 100 | 8 | 2 | 0 | 6 |
| Chicken or Turkey, fat free | 2 slices | 60 | 1 | 3 | 0 | 8 |
| Bouillon  - see Soup | ... | ... | . | . | . | . |
| Bratwurst, Boars Head | 1 wurst | 300 | 25 | 0 | 0 | 19 |
| Braunschweiger, 2 avg slices | 2 oz | 205 | 18 | 2 | Tr | 8 |
| **BREAD** | ... | ... | . | . | . | . |
| (½" thick slice unless noted) | ... | ... | . | . | . | . |
| Banana bread,  1 ¼" slice | 1 slice | 195 | 6 | 33 | 1 | 3 |
| Boston brown | 1 slice | 88 | 1 | 20 | 2 | 2 |
| Bran'ola | 1 slice | 90 | 2 | 18 | 2 | 3 |
| Bun, frankfurter, 1.4 oz, 5" long | 1 bun | 100 | 2 | 18 | 2 | 3 |
| Bun, hamburger, 1.4 oz | 1 bun | 100 | 2 | 18 | 2 | 3 |
| Bun, Lg, 7" long or  4" diameter | 1 bun | 200 | 4 | 36 | 4 | 6 |
| Carb Style, Pepperidge Farms | 1 slice | 60 | 2 | 8 | 3 | 5 |
| Carrot bread | 1 slice | 200 | 9 | 28 | 2 | 3 |
| Cinnamon raisin bread | 1 slice | 90 | 2 | 18 | 2 | 2 |
| Cornbread,  3" x  2" | 1 piece | 185 | 6 | 29 | 1 | 4 |
| Cracked wheat bread | 1 slice | 65 | 1 | 12 | 1 | 2 |
| Croissant, butter flavor, 4" | 1 | 230 | 12 | 26 | 2 | 5 |
| Egg bread, ¾" slice | 1 slice | 115 | 2 | 19 | 1 | 4 |
| English muffin, regular | 1 whole | 135 | 1 | 26 | 2 | 4 |
| English muffin, cinnamon/raisin | 1 whole | 140 | 2 | 28 | 2 | 4 |
| French bread | 1 slice | 70 | 1 | 13 | 1 | 2 |
| Garlic bread, ¾" thick | 1 slice | 150 | 8 | 16 | 1 | 3 |
| Italian bread | 1 slice | 65 | 1 | 12 | 1 | 2 |
| Multigrain bread | 1 slice | 65 | 1 | 12 | 2 | 3 |
| Oat/Oatmeal bread | 1 slice | 73 | 1 | 13 | 1 | 2 |
| Pita bread, 4" pita | 1 whole | 77 | Tr | 16 | 1 | 3 |
| Pita bread, 6 ½" pita | 1 whole | 165 | 1 | 33 | 1 | 5 |
| Potato bread | 1 slice | 100 | 2 | 18 | 2 | 3 |
| Pumpernickel bread | 1 slice | 80 | 1 | 15 | 2 | 3 |
| Raisin bread | 1 slice | 100 | 1 | 19 | 2 | 3 |
| Reduced calorie bread | 1 slice | 45 | Tr | 10 | 2 | 2 |
| Roll, cinnamon, w/glaze, 3" dia | 1 roll | 200 | 7 | 33 | 1 | 4 |
| Roll, hard or kaiser | 1 roll | 170 | 2 | 30 | 1 | 6 |
| Roll, soft, avg size, 1.4 oz | 1 roll | 100 | 1 | 18 | 2 | 2 |
| Rye bread | 1 slice | 75 | 1 | 14 | 2 | 3 |
| Sourdough bread | 1 slice | 70 | 1 | 13 | 1 | 2 |
| Submarine bread, 7" long | 1 | 200 | 4 | 36 | 4 | 6 |
| Vienna bread | 1 slice | 70 | 1 | 13 | 1 | 2 |

| FOOD: (See Beverages & Fast Food Restaurants listed separately) | Serving Size | Calories | Fat (g) | Carb (g) | Fiber (g) | Protein (g) |
|---|---|---|---|---|---|---|
| Wheat bread | 1 slice | 65 | 1 | 12 | 1 | 2 |
| White bread | 1 slice | 65 | 1 | 12 | 1 | 2 |
| White or Wheat, light bread | 1 slice | 45 | Tr | 10 | 2 | 2 |
| (also see Bagel & Biscuit) | ... | ... | . | . | . | . |
| Bread Crumbs | ... | ... | . | . | . | . |
| Dry, grated | 1 cup | 430 | 6 | 78 | 3 | 14 |
| Dry, seasoned, grated | 1 cup | 440 | 3 | 84 | 5 | 17 |
| Soft crumbs | 1 cup | 120 | 2 | 22 | 2 | 4 |
| Bread Stick | ... | ... | . | . | . | . |
| Crunchy w/sesame seeds, 0.4 oz | 1 | 40 | 1 | 7 | 1 | 1 |
| Soft, pizza flavored, 1.5 oz | 1 | 130 | 4 | 20 | 1 | 3 |
| Bread Stuffing – see Stuffing or | ... | ... | . | . | . | . |
| Bread Crumbs | ... | ... | . | . | . | . |
| Breakfast Sandwich, bacon, egg, | ... | ... | . | . | . | . |
| & cheese on English muffin | 1 avg | 370 | 28 | 19 | 2 | 15 |
| (also see Biscuit sandwiches) | ... | ... | . | . | . | . |
| Broccoli | ... | ... | . | . | . | . |
| Fresh, raw, flowerets | 3 | 9 | Tr | 3 | 1 | Tr |
| Fresh, raw, spear, 5" long | 1 | 9 | Tr | 2 | 1 | 1 |
| Fresh, raw, chopped or diced | 1 cup | 25 | Tr | 5 | 3 | 3 |
| Fresh, cooked, spear, 5" long | 1 | 10 | Tr | 2 | 1 | 1 |
| Fresh, chopped, cooked | 1 cup | 44 | 1 | 8 | 5 | 5 |
| Frozen, flowerets & cuts, cooked | 1 cup | 52 | Tr | 10 | 6 | 6 |
| Prep w/ butter sauce | ½ cup | 75 | 5 | 6 | 3 | 2 |
| Broccoli & Rice Casserole | ¾ cup | 240 | 12 | 26 | 5 | 5 |
| Broccoli Au gratin | ½ cup | 100 | 4 | 10 | 3 | 5 |
| Broth  - see Soup | ... | ... | . | . | . | . |
| Brownie, 2" square | ... | ... | . | . | . | . |
| With frosting | 1 | 190 | 8 | 27 | 1 | 2 |
| Without frosting | 1 | 140 | 6 | 20 | 1 | 2 |
| Fat Free | 1 | 90 | Tr | 22 | 1 | 1 |
| Brussels Sprouts | ... | ... | . | . | . | . |
| Fresh, cooked | 1 cup | 61 | 1 | 14 | 4 | 4 |
| Frozen, cooked | 1 cup | 65 | 1 | 13 | 6 | 6 |
| Prep w/ butter | ½ cup | 75 | 3 | 8 | 3 | 3 |
| Bugles  (snacks) | ... | ... | . | . | . | . |
| Regular | 1 ¼ cup | 150 | 7 | 20 | 1 | 1 |
| Baked | 1 ¼ cup | 130 | 4 | 23 | 1 | 2 |
| Nacho | 1 ¼ cup | 160 | 9 | 18 | 1 | 2 |
| Ranch | 1 ¼ cup | 160 | 9 | 18 | 1 | 2 |
| Sour cream & onion | 1 ¼ cup | 160 | 9 | 20 | 1 | 2 |

| FOOD:<br>(See Beverages & Fast Food<br>Restaurants listed separately) | Serv-ing Size | Cal-ories | Fat (g) | Carb (g) | Fi-ber (g) | Pro-tein (g) |
|---|---|---|---|---|---|---|
| Bulgur | ... | ... | . | . | . | . |
|   Cooked | 1 cup | 150 | Tr | 34 | 8 | 6 |
|   Uncooked | 1 cup | 480 | 2 | 106 | 26 | 17 |
| Bun - see Bread | ... | ... | . | . | . | . |
| Burrito | ... | ... | . | . | . | . |
|   Bean & cheese | 1 | 275 | 15 | 25 | 2 | 10 |
|   Bean & green chili | 1 | 270 | 9 | 35 | 3 | 10 |
|   Beans & rice | 1 | 200 | 3 | 36 | 2 | 6 |
|   Beef & bean | 1 | 300 | 17 | 26 | 2 | 11 |
|   Beef & cheese | 1 | 300 | 18 | 26 | 2 | 10 |
|   Chicken | 1 | 260 | 10 | 28 | 2 | 7 |
| Butter  (also see margarine) | ... | ... | . | . | . | . |
|   Regular stick, 4 sticks/pound | 1 stick | 815 | 92 | Tr | 0 | 1 |
|   Regular, salted or unsalted | 1 Tbsp | 100 | 12 | Tr | 0 | Tr |
|   Regular, salted or unsalted | 1 tsp | 34 | 4 | Tr | 0 | Tr |
|   Apple Butter | 1 Tbsp | 30 | 0 | 7 | Tr | Tr |
| Cabbage | ... | ... | . | . | . | . |
|   Green, raw, shredded | 1 cup | 18 | Tr | 4 | 2 | 1 |
|   Green, chopped, cooked | 1 cup | 33 | 1 | 7 | 4 | 2 |
|   Chinese cabbage (bok choy) | ... | ... | . | . | . | . |
|     shredded, raw | 1 cup | 10 | Tr | 2 | 2 | 1 |
|     shredded, cooked | 1 cup | 20 | Tr | 3 | 3 | 3 |
|   Red cabbage, raw, shredded | 1 cup | 19 | Tr | 4 | 1 | 1 |
|   Savoy cabbage, raw, shredded | 1 cup | 19 | Tr | 4 | 2 | 1 |
| Cabbage, Stuffed w/ beef or pork | 1 avg | 100 | 3 | 9 | 2 | 6 |
| CAKE | ... | ... | . | . | . | . |
|   (average slice of single layer | ... | ... | . | . | . | . |
|   cake, 1/8 of 9", unless noted) | ... | ... | . | . | . | . |
|   Angelfood cake, w/o frosting, | 1 piece | 125 | Tr | 28 | Tr | 3 |
|   Boston Cream Cake | 1 piece | 230 | 8 | 39 | 1 | 2 |
|   Carrot Cake, cream cheese icing | 1 piece | 485 | 29 | 52 | 2 | 5 |
|   Cheesecake, 1/6 of 17 oz cake | 1 piece | 260 | 18 | 20 | Tr | 5 |
|   Cheesecake w/chocolate | 1 piece | 580 | 41 | 44 | 1 | 9 |
|   Chocolate Cake | ... | ... | . | . | . | . |
|     w/frosting | 1 piece | 390 | 13 | 70 | 2 | 5 |
|     w/o frosting | 1 piece | 290 | 11 | 44 | 2 | 5 |
|   Coffee Crumb Cake, 2.2 oz | 1 piece | 265 | 15 | 29 | 1 | 4 |
|   Cupcake – see Cupcakes | ... | ... | . | . | . | . |
|   Devil's Food cake w/frosting | 1 piece | 395 | 13 | 71 | 2 | 5 |
|   Fat Free Cake, | ... | ... | . | . | . | . |
|     w/o frosting | 1 piece | 80 | Tr | 17 | Tr | 2 |

| FOOD: (See Beverages & Fast Food Restaurants listed separately) | Serv- ing Size | Cal- ories | Fat (g) | Carb (g) | Fi- ber (g) | Pro- tein (g) |
|---|---|---|---|---|---|---|
| w/sugar free glaze | 1 piece | 85 | Tr | 18 | Tr | 2 |
| Fruitcake, small slice | 1 piece | 160 | 5 | 27 | 2 | 1 |
| Gingerbread | 1 piece | 265 | 12 | 36 | 1 | 3 |
| Hummingbird | 1 piece | 595 | 30 | 72 | 1 | 5 |
| Marble cake, w/o frosting | 1 piece | 255 | 12 | 34 | 1 | 3 |
| Pineapple Upside Down Cake | 1 piece | 365 | 14 | 58 | 1 | 4 |
| Pound Cake w/o glaze | 1 piece | 220 | 11 | 29 | Tr | 3 |
| Shortcake, 3" dia | 1 piece | 225 | 9 | 32 | 1 | 4 |
| Sponge Cake | 1 piece | 180 | 3 | 35 | Tr | 5 |
| White Cake, | … | … | · | · | · | · |
| w/frosting | 1 piece | 395 | 12 | 71 | 1 | 5 |
| w/o frosting | 1 piece | 265 | 9 | 42 | 1 | 4 |
| Yellow Cake, | … | … | · | · | · | · |
| w/frosting | 1 piece | 390 | 12 | 70 | 1 | 5 |
| w/o frosting | 1 piece | 260 | 9 | 42 | 1 | 4 |
| **CANDY & Chocolate Bars** | … | … | · | · | · | · |
| Atomic FireBall, ¾" dia | 1 | 24 | 0 | 6 | 0 | 0 |
| Almond Joy, 1.7 oz bar | 1 bar | 240 | 13 | 29 | 2 | 2 |
| Baby Ruth, 2.1 oz bar | 1 bar | 290 | 13 | 39 | 1 | 5 |
| Bit-O-Honey, 2.1 oz | 1 bar | 185 | 4 | 39 | Tr | 1 |
| BreathSavers, sugar free | 1 | 5 | 0 | 2 | 0 | 0 |
| Butterfinger, 2.1 oz bar | 1 bar | 280 | 8 | 41 | 2 | 8 |
| Candy Cane, 0.5 oz | 1 cane | 55 | 0 | 14 | 0 | 0 |
| Candy Corn | ¼ cup | 180 | 1 | 45 | 0 | 0 |
| Caramel | … | … | · | · | · | · |
| regular caramel, 0.3 oz | 1 piece | 35 | 1 | 7 | Tr | Tr |
| regular caramel, 2.5 oz | 2.5 oz | 270 | 6 | 55 | 1 | 3 |
| chocolate caramel, 0.3 oz | 1 piece | 25 | Tr | 6 | Tr | Tr |
| Carob | 1 oz | 155 | 9 | 16 | 1 | 2 |
| Charms Blow Pop | 1 | 60 | 0 | 14 | 0 | 0 |
| Chewing Gum-see separately | … | … | · | · | · | · |
| Chocolate Bars | … | … | · | · | · | · |
| Hershey's Chocolate bar, | … | … | · | · | · | · |
| plain, 1.5 oz bar | 1 bar | 230 | 13 | 25 | 1 | 3 |
| Hershey's Nugget, 10g | 1 bar | 52 | 3 | 6 | Tr | 1 |
| Hershey's Snack Size, 17g | 1 bar | 90 | 5 | 10 | Tr | 1 |
| with almonds, 1.45 oz | 1 bar | 220 | 14 | 22 | 3 | 4 |
| with crispy rice, 1.55 oz | 1 bar | 230 | 12 | 29 | 1 | 3 |
| with peanuts, 1.75 oz | 1 bar | 265 | 17 | 25 | 2 | 5 |
| (see 'Chocolate for Baking' | … | … | · | · | · | · |
| listed separately) | … | … | · | · | · | · |

| FOOD: (See Beverages & Fast Food Restaurants listed separately) | Serv- ing Size | Cal- ories | Fat (g) | Carb (g) | Fi- ber (g) | Pro- tein (g) |
|---|---|---|---|---|---|---|
| Chocolate Coated Peanuts | 10 | 205 | 13 | 20 | 2 | 5 |
| Chocolate Coated Raisins | 10 | 40 | 1 | 7 | 2 | Tr |
| Chocolate Kiss, Hershey's | 4 | 102 | 6 | 11 | Tr | 1 |
| Fifth Avenue bar, 2 oz | 1 bar | 195 | 8 | 26 | 1 | 4 |
| Fruit Leather Bar | 1 oz | 95 | 2 | 22 | 1 | Tr |
| Fruit Leather, small roll | 1 roll | 50 | Tr | 12 | 1 | Tr |
| Fudge, chocolate, 0.6 oz piece | 1 piece | 65 | 1 | 13 | 1 | Tr |
| Goobers, 1.4 oz | 1 | 200 | 13 | 6 | 0 | 5 |
| Gumdrops ¾" dia | 5 | 64 | 0 | 16 | 0 | 0 |
| Gummy Bears | 10 | 85 | 0 | 22 | 0 | 0 |
| Gummy Worms | 10 | 285 | 0 | 73 | 0 | 0 |
| Hard Candy, regular, 1" dia | ... | ... | . | . | . | . |
| Butterscotch or Coffee flavor | 2 | 42 | 0 | 10 | 0 | 0 |
| Cinnamon, Fruit, Mint flavor | 2 | 40 | 0 | 10 | 0 | 0 |
| Hard Candy, sugar free | ... | ... | . | . | . | . |
| Baskin Robbins, sugarfree | ... | ... | . | . | . | . |
| Fruit or Chocolate Mint | 2 | 20 | 1 | 7 | 0 | 0 |
| Brachs, sugar free Cinnamon | 3 | 35 | 0 | 17 | 0 | 0 |
| Life Savers, sugar free | 4 | 30 | 0 | 14 | 0 | 0 |
| Sweet 'N Low Fruit Flavors | 5 | 30 | 0 | 14 | 0 | 0 |
| Sweet 'N Low Butterscotch | 5 | 30 | 0 | 15 | 0 | 0 |
| Sweet 'N Low Coffee | 5 | 30 | 0 | 14 | 0 | 0 |
| Jawbreaker, regular size, ¾" dia | 1 | 24 | 0 | 6 | 0 | 0 |
| Jawbreaker, large size, 1" dia | 1 | 40 | 0 | 9 | 0 | 0 |
| Jelly Beans, regular size | 10 | 100 | Tr | 25 | 0 | 0 |
| Jelly Beans, small pieces | 10 | 40 | Tr | 10 | 0 | 0 |
| Kit Kat bar, 1.5 oz | 1 bar | 215 | 11 | 27 | Tr | 3 |
| Krackel bar, 1.5 oz | 1 bar | 220 | 12 | 25 | 1 | 3 |
| Licorice, 1.4 oz pkg | 1.4 oz | 135 | 1 | 31 | 0 | 1 |
| LifeSavers | 2 | 20 | 0 | 5 | 0 | 0 |
| Lollipop, Charms Blow Pop 15g | 1 | 60 | 0 | 14 | 0 | 0 |
| Lollipop, large, 14 g | 1 | 50 | 0 | 12 | 0 | 0 |
| Lollipop, small, Dum Dum, 5 g | 1 | 24 | 0 | 6 | 0 | 0 |
| M&M candy, plain | 10 | 34 | 1 | 5 | Tr | Tr |
| M&M candy, w/ nuts | 10 | 103 | 5 | 12 | 1 | 2 |
| Mars Almond bar, 1.75 oz | 1 bar | 235 | 12 | 31 | 2 | 4 |
| Marshmallow, avg size | 1 | 23 | 0 | 6 | 0 | 0 |
| Milky Way, reg size, 2.15 oz | 1 bar | 258 | 10 | 44 | 1 | 3 |
| Milky Way, small, fun size | 1 bar | 76 | 3 | 13 | Tr | 1 |
| Mints, pastel, ½" square | 10 | 75 | 0 | 18 | 0 | 0 |
| Mounds, 1.9 oz bar | 1 bar | 255 | 13 | 31 | 2 | 2 |

| FOOD: (See Beverages & Fast Food Restaurants listed separately) | Serving Size | Calories | Fat (g) | Carb (g) | Fiber (g) | Protein (g) |
|---|---|---|---|---|---|---|
| Mr. Goodbar, 1.75 oz | 1 bar | 265 | 17 | 25 | 2 | 5 |
| Oh Henry, 2 oz bar | 1 bar | 245 | 10 | 37 | 1 | 6 |
| Nestle Crunch bar, 1.55 oz | 1 bar | 230 | 12 | 29 | 1 | 3 |
| Peanut Brittle | 1 oz | 130 | 5 | 20 | 1 | 2 |
| Peppermint Pattie, 1.5 oz | 1 pattie | 165 | 3 | 34 | 1 | 1 |
| Raisinets, 1.6 oz pkg | 1 pkg | 185 | 7 | 32 | 6 | 2 |
| Reese's Peanut Butter Cups | … | … | . | . | . | . |
|   regular size cups | 2 cups | 245 | 14 | 25 | 1 | 5 |
|   miniature size cups | 2 cups | 42 | 2 | 4 | Tr | 1 |
| Reese's Pieces, 1.6 oz pkg | 1 pkg | 225 | 9 | 28 | 1 | 6 |
| Reese Sticks, 0.6 oz bar | 1 bar | 90 | 1 | 9 | Tr | 2 |
| Rolo caramels | 9 piece | 220 | 11 | 28 | 1 | 3 |
| Skittles, 2.3 oz pkg | 1 pkg | 265 | 3 | 59 | Tr | 0 |
| Skor toffee bar, 1.4 oz | 1 bar | 220 | 2 | 23 | Tr | 13 |
| Snickers bar, regular size, 2 oz | 1 bar | 275 | 14 | 34 | 1 | 5 |
| Snickers bar, small fun size | 1 bar | 72 | 4 | 9 | Tr | 1 |
| Special Dark, miniature bar | 1 bar | 46 | 3 | 5 | Tr | Tr |
| Starburst Fruit Chews, 2 oz pkg | 1 pkg | 235 | 5 | 50 | 0 | Tr |
| Starlight Mints, 1" dia | 3 | 56 | 0 | 14 | 0 | 0 |
| Sucker – see Lollipop | … | … | . | . | . | . |
| Three Musketeers, 2.1 oz bar | 1 bar | 250 | 8 | 46 | Tr | 2 |
| Toffee, 1.4 oz bar | 1 bar | 220 | 13 | 23 | 1 | 2 |
| Tootsie Roll, 1 oz | 1 oz | 110 | 6 | 15 | Tr | 1 |
| Twizzlers, Cherry, 2.5 oz pkg | 1 pkg | 135 | 1 | 31 | 0 | 1 |
| Cannelloni, Cheese | … | … | . | . | . | . |
|   Lean Cuisine entrée | 1 meal | 250 | 6 | 30 | 2 | 16 |
| Cantaloupe | … | … | . | . | . | . |
|   Fresh, medium size, 5" dia | ½ | 98 | Tr | 22 | 2 | 3 |
|   Fresh, wedge 1/8 melon | 1 wedge | 25 | Tr | 6 | 1 | 1 |
|   Fresh, cubed | 1 cup | 55 | Tr | 13 | 1 | 1 |
| Carambola (starfruit) | … | … | . | . | . | . |
|   Fresh, 3 ½", whole | 1 | 30 | Tr | 7 | 3 | Tr |
|   Fresh, sliced | 1 cup | 36 | Tr | 8 | 3 | 1 |
| Caramels – see candy | … | … | . | . | . | . |
| Carrot | … | … | . | . | . | . |
|   Fresh, raw, whole, 7 ½" long | 1 | 32 | Tr | 7 | 2 | 1 |
|   Fresh, raw, shredded | 1 cup | 47 | Tr | 11 | 3 | 1 |
|   Fresh, baby carrots | 2 | 12 | Tr | 3 | 1 | Tr |
|   Fresh, cooked, slices | 1 cup | 65 | Tr | 14 | 5 | 2 |
|   Frozen, cooked, slices | 1 cup | 69 | Tr | 15 | 5 | 2 |
|   Canned, drained, slices, cooked | 1 cup | 57 | Tr | 13 | 3 | 1 |

| FOOD: (See Beverages & Fast Food Restaurants listed separately) | Serv-ing Size | Cal-ories | Fat (g) | Carb (g) | Fi-ber (g) | Pro-tein (g) |
|---|---|---|---|---|---|---|
| Glazed carrots | ¾ cup | 280 | 15 | 35 | 5 | 1 |
| Cashew – see Nuts | ... | ... | . | . | . | . |
| Casserole, see specific listings | ... | ... | . | . | . | . |
| Catsup, regular | 1 Tbsp | 18 | Tr | 4 | Tr | Tr |
|    Restaurant size packet | 1 pkt | 10 | Tr | 3 | Tr | Tr |
| Cauliflower | ... | ... | . | . | . | . |
|    Fresh, raw, flowerets | 3 | 9 | Tr | 3 | 1 | Tr |
|    Fresh, raw, chopped or diced | 1 cup | 25 | Tr | 5 | 3 | 2 |
|    Fresh, flowerets, cooked | 3 | 12 | Tr | 2 | 1 | 1 |
|    Fresh, chopped, cooked | 1 cup | 30 | Tr | 5 | 3 | 2 |
|    Frozen, cuts, cooked | 1 cup | 35 | Tr | 7 | 5 | 3 |
|    Prep w/ butter | ¾ cup | 100 | 8 | 6 | 2 | 2 |
|    Prep w/ cheese sauce | ¾ cup | 110 | 8 | 6 | 2 | 4 |
| Cavatelli | 1 cup | 400 | 2 | 77 | 1 | 14 |
| Caviar – see Fish | ... | ... | . | . | . | . |
| Cayenne, dried spice | ¼ tsp | 1 | 0 | Tr | Tr | Tr |
| Caesar Salad | 4 oz | 200 | 17 | 7 | 2 | 7 |
| Celery | ... | ... | . | . | . | . |
|    Fresh, raw, stalk, 7 ½" long | 1 stalk | 6 | Tr | 1 | Tr | Tr |
|    Fresh, raw, diced | 1 cup | 19 | Tr | 4 | 2 | 1 |
|    Cooked, stalk 7 ½" long | 1 stalk | 6 | Tr | 1 | Tr | Tr |
|    Cooked, diced pieces | 1 cup | 27 | Tr | 6 | 2 | 1 |
| Celery Seed | 1 tsp | 8 | 1 | 1 | Tr | Tr |
| **CEREAL** | ... | ... | . | . | . | . |
|    All-Bran | ½ cup | 80 | 1 | 23 | 10 | 4 |
|    Apple Jacks | 1 cup | 116 | Tr | 27 | 1 | 1 |
|    Cap'n Crunch, regular | ¾ cup | 107 | 1 | 23 | 1 | 1 |
|       Crunchberries | ¾ cup | 104 | 1 | 22 | 1 | 1 |
|       Peanut Butter Crunchy | ¾ cup | 112 | 2 | 22 | 1 | 2 |
|    Cheerios Cereal, regular | 1 cup | 110 | 2 | 23 | 3 | 3 |
|       Apple Cinnamon Cheerios | ¾ cup | 118 | 2 | 25 | 2 | 2 |
|    Chex Cereal, Corn | 1 cup | 113 | Tr | 26 | 1 | 2 |
|       Honey Nut | ¾ cup | 117 | 1 | 26 | Tr | 2 |
|       Multi Bran | 1 cup | 170 | 1 | 39 | 5 | 4 |
|       Rice | 1¼ cup | 117 | Tr | 27 | Tr | 2 |
|       Wheat | 1 cup | 104 | 1 | 24 | 3 | 3 |
|    Cinnamon Toast Crunch | ¾ cup | 124 | 3 | 24 | 2 | 2 |
|    Cocoa Krispies | ¾ cup | 120 | 1 | 27 | Tr | 2 |
|    Cocoa Puffs | 1 cup | 120 | 1 | 27 | Tr | 1 |
|    Corn Flakes | 1 cup | 105 | Tr | 24 | 1 | 2 |
|    Corn Pops | 1 cup | 118 | Tr | 28 | Tr | 1 |

| FOOD: (See Beverages & Fast Food Restaurants listed separately) | Serving Size | Calories | Fat (g) | Carb (g) | Fiber (g) | Protein (g) |
|---|---|---|---|---|---|---|
| Cream of Wheat, as prep | 1 cup | 130 | Tr | 27 | 1 | 4 |
| Crispix | 1 cup | 108 | Tr | 25 | 1 | 2 |
| Fruit Loops | 1 cup | 117 | 1 | 26 | 1 | 1 |
| Frosted Flakes | 1 cup | 120 | Tr | 28 | 1 | 1 |
| Frosted Mini Wheats | ... | ... | . | . | . | . |
|   regular size | 1 cup | 175 | 1 | 42 | 6 | 5 |
|   bite size | 1 cup | 190 | 1 | 45 | 6 | 5 |
| Golden Grahams | ¾ cup | 116 | 1 | 26 | 1 | 2 |
| Granola Cereal, Nature Valley | ¾ cup | 250 | 10 | 36 | 4 | 6 |
| Honey Nut Cheerios | 1 cup | 115 | 1 | 24 | 2 | 3 |
| Kix Cereal, regular | 1¼ cup | 114 | 1 | 26 | 1 | 2 |
|   Kix Berry Berry | ¾ cup | 120 | 1 | 26 | Tr | 1 |
| Life Cereal, regular | ¾ cup | 120 | 1 | 25 | 2 | 3 |
|   Life Cinnamon Cereal | 1 cup | 190 | 2 | 40 | 3 | 4 |
| Lucky Charms | 1 cup | 116 | 1 | 25 | 1 | 2 |
| Malt O Meal, as prep | 1 cup | 122 | Tr | 26 | 1 | 4 |
| Oat Cereal, Cheerios type | 1 cup | 110 | 2 | 23 | 3 | 3 |
| Oatmeal, warm - see Oatmeal | ... | ... | . | . | . | . |
| Peanut Butter Puffed Cereal | ¾ cup | 130 | 3 | 23 | Tr | 3 |
| Product 19 | 1 cup | 110 | Tr | 25 | 1 | 3 |
| Puffed Rice Cereal | 1 cup | 56 | Tr | 13 | Tr | 1 |
| Puffed Wheat Cereal | 1 cup | 44 | Tr | 10 | 1 | 2 |
| Raisin Bran Cereal | 1 cup | 180 | 1 | 45 | 7 | 1 |
| Raisin Nut Bran | 1 cup | 210 | 4 | 41 | 5 | 5 |
| Rice Crispies | 1¼ cup | 124 | Tr | 29 | Tr | 2 |
| Shredded wheat cereal, | ... | ... | . | . | . | . |
|   frosted biscuits | 1 cup | 190 | 1 | 45 | 6 | 5 |
| Smacks Cereal | ¾ cup | 105 | Tr | 24 | 1 | 2 |
| Special K | 1 cup | 115 | Tr | 22 | 1 | 6 |
| Total | ¾ cup | 105 | 1 | 24 | 3 | 3 |
| Trix Cereal | 1 cup | 122 | 2 | 26 | 1 | 1 |
| Wheat Bran Flakes | ¾ cup | 95 | 1 | 23 | 5 | 3 |
| Wheaties | 1 cup | 110 | 1 | 24 | 2 | 3 |
| Cereal Bar | ... | ... | . | . | . | . |
|   Granola Chocolate Chip-small | 1 bar | 90 | 2 | 19 | 1 | 1 |
|   Plain- regular size bar | 1 bar | 135 | 2 | 28 | 1 | 2 |
|   Fruit filled- regular size bar | 1 bar | 145 | 2 | 29 | 1 | 2 |
| Chalupa | ... | ... | . | . | . | . |
|   Beef | 1 | 380 | 23 | 29 | 2 | 14 |
|   Chicken | 1 | 360 | 20 | 28 | 2 | 17 |
|   Nacho cheese & beef | 1 | 370 | 22 | 30 | 2 | 13 |

| FOOD: (See Beverages & Fast Food Restaurants listed separately) | Serving Size | Calories | Fat (g) | Carb (g) | Fiber (g) | Protein (g) |
|---|---|---|---|---|---|---|
| Nacho cheese & chicken | 1 | 350 | 19 | 29 | 2 | 16 |
| Nacho cheese & steak | 1 | 350 | 19 | 28 | 2 | 16 |
| **CHEESE** | ... | ... | . | . | . | . |
| American, pasteurized cheese | ... | ... | . | . | . | . |
| regular | 1 oz | 105 | 9 | 1 | 0 | 6 |
| fat free | 1 slice | 25 | 0 | 3 | 0 | 4 |
| Blue cheese | 1 oz | 100 | 8 | 1 | 0 | 6 |
| Camembert 1.3 oz | 1 pc | 114 | 9 | Tr | 0 | 8 |
| Cheddar cheese | ... | ... | . | . | . | . |
| regular, 1 ounce slice | 1 slice | 115 | 9 | Tr | 0 | 7 |
| 1 inch cube | 1 slice | 68 | 6 | Tr | 0 | 4 |
| shredded | 1 cup | 455 | 37 | 1 | 0 | 28 |
| lowfat | 1 oz | 50 | 2 | 1 | 0 | 7 |
| fat free | 1 slice | 25 | 0 | 3 | 0 | 4 |
| Cheese food, pasteurized | 1 oz | 93 | 7 | 2 | 0 | 6 |
| Cheese spread, pasteurized | 1 oz | 82 | 6 | 2 | 0 | 5 |
| Colby cheese | 1 oz | 112 | 9 | 1 | 0 | 7 |
| Cottage cheese | ... | ... | . | . | . | . |
| regular, creamed, 4% fat | ... | ... | . | . | . | . |
| large curd | 1 cup | 233 | 10 | 6 | 0 | 28 |
| small curd | 1 cup | 217 | 9 | 6 | 0 | 26 |
| with fruit | 1 cup | 279 | 8 | 30 | 0 | 22 |
| lowfat, 2% fat | 1 cup | 203 | 4 | 8 | 0 | 31 |
| lowfat, 1% fat | 1 cup | 164 | 2 | 6 | 0 | 28 |
| fat free | 1 cup | 160 | 0 | 10 | 0 | 30 |
| dry curd, uncreamed, 0.5% fat | 1 cup | 123 | 1 | 3 | 0 | 25 |
| Cream cheese | ... | ... | . | . | . | . |
| regular cream | 1 oz | 100 | 10 | 1 | 0 | 2 |
| regular cream | 1 Tbsp | 50 | 5 | Tr | 0 | 1 |
| lowfat/light | 1 Tbsp | 35 | 3 | 1 | 0 | 2 |
| fat free | 1 Tbsp | 15 | 0 | 1 | 0 | 2 |
| Feta cheese | 1 oz | 75 | 6 | 1 | 0 | 4 |
| Fontina cheese | 1 oz | 110 | 9 | 1 | 0 | 7 |
| Goat cheese, soft | 1 oz | 75 | 6 | 1 | 0 | 4 |
| Jalapeno jack cheese | 1 oz | 90 | 8 | 1 | 0 | 5 |
| Monterey jack cheese | 1 oz | 105 | 9 | Tr | 0 | 7 |
| Mozzarella cheese | ... | ... | . | . | . | . |
| regular, 1 ounce slice | 1 slice | 80 | 5 | 1 | 0 | 8 |
| shredded, 2 oz | ½ cup | 160 | 10 | 2 | 0 | 16 |
| fat free | 1 slice | 25 | 0 | 3 | 0 | 4 |
| Muenster cheese, sliced | 1 oz | 105 | 9 | Tr | 0 | 7 |

| FOOD: (See Beverages & Fast Food Restaurants listed separately) | Serving Size | Calories | Fat (g) | Carb (g) | Fiber (g) | Protein (g) |
|---|---|---|---|---|---|---|
| Neufchatel cheese | 1 oz | 75 | 7 | 1 | 0 | 3 |
| Parmesan cheese | ... | ... | . | . | . | . |
| grated, 1 cup | 1 cup | 455 | 30 | 4 | 0 | 42 |
| grated, 1 tablespoon | 1 Tbsp | 25 | 2 | Tr | 0 | 2 |
| Provolone cheese | 1 oz | 100 | 8 | 1 | 0 | 7 |
| Ricotta cheese | ... | ... | . | . | . | . |
| regular | 1 cup | 430 | 32 | 7 | 0 | 28 |
| part skim | 1 cup | 340 | 19 | 13 | 0 | 28 |
| fat free | 1 cup | 240 | 0 | 20 | 0 | 40 |
| Romano cheese, grated | 1 oz | 110 | 8 | 1 | 0 | 9 |
| Roquefort, sheep's milk | 1 oz | 105 | 9 | 1 | 0 | 6 |
| Swiss cheese | ... | ... | . | . | . | . |
| regular, 1 ounce slice | 1 slice | 105 | 8 | 1 | 0 | 8 |
| fat free | 1 slice | 25 | 0 | 3 | 0 | 4 |
| Cheeseburger (see hamburger) | ... | ... | . | . | . | . |
| Cheese Puffs (about 25) | 1 oz | 160 | 10 | 15 | Tr | 2 |
| Cheese Puffs Balls (2 ½ cups) | 1 oz | 160 | 10 | 15 | Tr | 2 |
| Cheese Spread | ... | ... | . | . | . | . |
| Cheez Whiz | 2 Tbsp | 90 | 7 | 2 | 0 | 5 |
| Velveeta | 2 Tbsp | 80 | 6 | 3 | 0 | 5 |
| Cheetos (snacks) | ... | ... | . | . | . | . |
| Curls (about 15) | 1 oz | 150 | 10 | 15 | Tr | 2 |
| Puffs (about 25) | 1 oz | 160 | 10 | 15 | Tr | 2 |
| Cherries | ... | ... | . | . | . | . |
| Fresh, sweet | 10 | 50 | 1 | 11 | 2 | 1 |
| Sour, canned, water pack | 1 cup | 90 | Tr | 22 | 3 | 2 |
| Cherry Pie Filling, canned | 3 oz | 80 | Tr | 20 | Tr | Tr |
| Chestnut – see Nuts | ... | ... | . | . | . | . |
| **Chewing Gum**, | ... | ... | . | . | . | . |
| Stick Gum, 2 ¾" long | ... | ... | . | . | . | . |
| Regular stick gum | 1 stick | 10 | 0 | 2 | 0 | 0 |
| Wrigley's Extra, sugarfree | 1 stick | 5 | 0 | 2 | 0 | 0 |
| Carefree, sugarfree | 1 stick | 5 | 0 | 2 | 0 | 0 |
| Bubble Yum, all regular flavors | 1 | 25 | 0 | 6 | 0 | 0 |
| Dentyne Ice, all flavors | 2 | 5 | 0 | 2 | 0 | 0 |
| Gum Balls, small, ½" dia balls | 5 | 40 | 0 | 10 | 0 | 0 |
| Gum Balls, Lg, 1 ¼" dia balls | 1 | 32 | 0 | 8 | 0 | 0 |
| Grapermelon, Wrigley's, ¾" | 2 | 10 | 0 | 2 | 0 | 0 |
| Strappleberry, Wrigley's , ¾" | 2 | 10 | 0 | 2 | 0 | 0 |
| Trident, all flavors, 1" sticks | 1 stick | 5 | 0 | 1 | 0 | 0 |
| Chex Mix, 1 oz | 2/3 cup | 120 | 5 | 18 | 2 | 3 |

| FOOD: (See Beverages & Fast Food Restaurants listed separately) | Serv-ing Size | Cal-ories | Fat (g) | Carb (g) | Fi-ber (g) | Pro-tein (g) |
|---|---|---|---|---|---|---|
| **CHICKEN** | ... | ... | . | . | . | . |
| Giblets, simmered, chopped | 1 cup | 230 | 7 | 1 | 0 | 37 |
| Fried Chicken, batter dipped | ... | ... | . | . | . | . |
| ½ Breast, about 4 oz | ½ | 365 | 18 | 13 | Tr | 35 |
| Drumstick, avg size | 1 | 195 | 11 | 6 | Tr | 16 |
| Thigh, avg size | 1 | 240 | 14 | 8 | Tr | 19 |
| Wing, avg size | 2 | 160 | 11 | 5 | Tr | 10 |
| Strips, dark meat | 3 oz | 205 | 9 | 10 | Tr | 25 |
| Strips, white meat | 3 oz | 175 | 5 | 7 | Tr | 25 |
| Liver of chicken, simmered | 1 | 31 | 1 | Tr | 0 | 5 |
| Neck, simmered | 1 | 32 | 1 | 0 | 0 | 4 |
| Roasted or Broiled Chicken | ... | ... | . | . | . | . |
| ½ Breast, about 3.5 oz meat | ½ | 165 | 4 | 0 | 0 | 32 |
| Drumstick, avg size | 1 | 75 | 2 | 0 | 0 | 12 |
| Thigh, avg size | 1 | 110 | 6 | 0 | 0 | 13 |
| White meat w/ skin | 3.5 oz | 280 | 12 | 0 | 0 | 33 |
| White meat, skinless | 3.5 oz | 170 | 4 | 0 | 0 | 33 |
| Dark meat w/ skin | 3.5 oz | 320 | 21 | 0 | 0 | 22 |
| Dark meat skinless | 3.5 oz | 190 | 10 | 0 | 0 | 22 |
| Canned, boneless | 5 oz | 235 | 11 | 0 | 0 | 31 |
| Stewed Chicken | ... | ... | . | . | . | . |
| Light & dark meat, diced | 1 cup | 330 | 17 | 0 | 0 | 43 |
| Wings, Buffalo, hot | 4 | 220 | 11 | 3 | 0 | 22 |
| Wings, skinless, unbreaded | 4 | 220 | 11 | 3 | 0 | 22 |
| (Other Chicken Products, see: | ... | ... | . | . | . | . |
| Bologna, Hot Dog, Salami, | ... | ... | . | . | . | . |
| Sausage & specific entrées) | ... | ... | . | . | . | . |
| Chicken a la King | 1 cup | 320 | 22 | 17 | Tr | 15 |
| Chicken Alfredo | 1 cup | 300 | 10 | 35 | Tr | 18 |
| Chicken & Broccoli Alfredo | 1 ½ cup | 300 | 6 | 38 | 1 | 25 |
| Chicken Cacciatoré | ... | ... | . | . | . | . |
| Healthy Choice entrée | 1 meal | 250 | 3 | 36 | 1 | 21 |
| Lean Cuisine entrée | 1 meal | 280 | 10 | 25 | 1 | 23 |
| Chicken Cordon Blue | ... | ... | . | . | . | . |
| Le Menu entrée | 1 meal | 460 | 20 | 48 | 1 | 23 |
| Chicken Dijon, Healthy Choice | 1 meal | 270 | 5 | 33 | 1 | 23 |
| Chicken Francesca | ... | ... | . | . | . | . |
| Healthy Choice entrée | 1 meal | 330 | 6 | 46 | 1 | 23 |
| Chicken Kiev, Tyson entrée | 1 meal | 440 | 25 | 36 | 1 | 18 |
| Chicken Marsala, Tyson entrée | 1 meal | 180 | 5 | 19 | 1 | 15 |
| Chicken Nuggets | ... | ... | . | . | . | . |

| FOOD:<br>(See Beverages & Fast Food Restaurants listed separately) | Serv-ing Size | Cal-ories | Fat (g) | Carb (g) | Fi-ber (g) | Pro-tein (g) |
|---|---|---|---|---|---|---|
| Banquet entrée | 1 meal | 410 | 21 | 38 | 1 | 18 |
| Morton entrée | 1 meal | 320 | 17 | 30 | 1 | 13 |
| Chicken Parmagiana | ... | ... | . | . | . | . |
| Banquet entrée | 1 meal | 290 | 15 | 27 | 1 | 14 |
| Healthy Choice entrée | 1 meal | 300 | 4 | 47 | 1 | 20 |
| Le Menu entrée | 1 meal | 395 | 19 | 30 | 1 | 26 |
| Chicken Roll, light meat | 2 oz | 90 | 4 | 2 | 1 | 11 |
| Chicken Teriyaki w/vegetables | 1 cup | 200 | 8 | 20 | 2 | 12 |
| Chicken w/Sweet & Sour Sauce | 1 cup | 320 | 5 | 53 | 2 | 19 |
| Chicken w/Vegetables | ... | ... | . | . | . | . |
| Lean Cuisine entrée | 1 meal | 250 | 5 | 33 | 2 | 18 |
| Chickpeas, cooked | ½ cup | 140 | 2 | 25 | 6 | 7 |
| Chili Powder | 1 tsp | 8 | Tr | 1 | Tr | Tr |
| Chili w/Beans | 1 cup | 270 | 11 | 23 | 8 | 21 |
| Chili Con Carne w/Beans | 1 cup | 255 | 8 | 24 | 8 | 20 |
| Chimichanga | ... | ... | . | . | . | . |
| Beans & cheese | 1 | 300 | 17 | 25 | 1 | 9 |
| Beef & cheese | 1 | 425 | 20 | 43 | 1 | 20 |
| Chicken & cheese | 1 | 350 | 16 | 39 | 1 | 11 |
| Chips – see Corn Chips, Potato | ... | ... | . | . | . | . |
| Chips & other specific listings | ... | ... | . | . | . | . |
| Chives, raw, chopped | 1 Tbsp | 1 | Tr | Tr | Tr | Tr |
| Chocolate for Baking (Also see | ... | ... | . | . | . | . |
| 'Candy' for other chocolates) | ... | ... | . | . | . | . |
| Chocolate Chips, milk, regular | 1 cup | 860 | 52 | 99 | 6 | 12 |
| Chocolate Chips, semisweet | 1 cup | 805 | 50 | 106 | 10 | 7 |
| Chocolate Chips, white | 1 cup | 915 | 55 | 101 | 0 | 10 |
| Unsweetened for baking, solid | 1 sq | 148 | 16 | 8 | 4 | 3 |
| Unsweetened, liquid | 1 oz | 134 | 14 | 10 | 5 | 3 |
| Chow Mein | ... | ... | . | . | . | . |
| Beef chow mein | 1 ½ cup | 170 | 6 | 12 | 2 | 14 |
| Chicken chow mein | 1 ½ cup | 160 | 7 | 12 | 2 | 14 |
| Cilantro, raw | 1 tsp | Tr | Tr | Tr | Tr | Tr |
| Cinnamon | 1 tsp | 6 | Tr | 2 | 1 | Tr |
| Cinnamon Sweet Roll | ... | ... | . | . | . | . |
| With glaze, 3" dia | 1 | 200 | 7 | 33 | 1 | 4 |
| With raisins & glaze, 3" dia | 1 | 225 | 10 | 35 | 1 | 4 |
| With raisins & glaze, 4 ½" dia | 1 | 510 | 15 | 85 | 2 | 8 |
| Clam Chowder - see Soup | ... | ... | . | . | . | . |
| Clams – see Fish/Seafood | ... | ... | . | . | . | . |

| FOOD: (See Beverages & Fast Food Restaurants listed separately) | Serving Size | Calories | Fat (g) | Carb (g) | Fiber (g) | Protein (g) |
|---|---|---|---|---|---|---|
| Cloves, ground | 1 tsp | 6 | Tr | 1 | Tr | Tr |
| Cocoa, unsweetened powder | 1 Tbsp | 15 | 1 | 3 | 2 | 1 |
| Cocoa, unsweetened, powder | 1 cup | 240 | 16 | 48 | 32 | 16 |
| Coconut | … | … | . | . | . | . |
| Fresh piece, 2" x 2" x ½" | 1 piece | 160 | 15 | 7 | 4 | 1 |
| Fresh, shredded, not packed | 1 cup | 285 | 27 | 12 | 7 | 3 |
| Dried, sweetened, flaked | 1 cup | 465 | 33 | 44 | 4 | 3 |
| Coleslaw | ½ cup | 62 | 2 | 10 | 1 | 1 |
| Collards | … | … | . | . | . | . |
| Fresh, chopped, cooked | 1 cup | 49 | 1 | 9 | 5 | 4 |
| Frozen, chopped, cooked | 1 cup | 61 | 1 | 12 | 5 | 5 |
| Condiments, see Sauce, | … | … | . | . | . | . |
| or see specific listing | … | … | . | . | . | . |
| **COOKIES** 2 ¼" diameter | … | … | . | . | . | . |
| unless noted | … | … | . | . | . | . |
| Animal Crackers, 1" dia | 8 | 60 | 1 | 12 | Tr | 1 |
| Butter Cookie | 1 | 50 | 2 | 7 | Tr | Tr |
| Chocolate Chip, regular | 1 | 80 | 3 | 12 | 1 | 2 |
| Chocolate Chip, reduced fat | 1 | 70 | 1 | 12 | 1 | 2 |
| Chocolate Chip, sugar free | 1 | 70 | 6 | 10 | 1 | 1 |
| Coconut cookie | 1 | 75 | 3 | 11 | 1 | 1 |
| Fig Newton | 2 | 110 | 2 | 20 | 1 | 1 |
| Molasses cookie | 1 | 80 | 2 | 13 | Tr | 1 |
| Oatmeal w/ raisins | 1 | 75 | 2 | 12 | 1 | 1 |
| Oatmeal, plain | 1 | 70 | 2 | 11 | 1 | 1 |
| Oatmeal, sugarfree | 1 | 70 | 6 | 10 | 1 | 1 |
| Peanut Butter, plain | 1 | 80 | 2 | 10 | Tr | 1 |
| Peanut Butter w/ nuts | 1 | 90 | 3 | 11 | Tr | 2 |
| Pecan Shortbread cookie | 1 | 75 | 5 | 8 | Tr | 1 |
| Sandwich cookie, w/ filling, | … | … | . | . | . | . |
| 1 ½" dia, round, | … | … | . | . | . | . |
| chocolate w/ creme filling | 1 | 50 | 2 | 7 | Tr | Tr |
| sugar w/ peanut butter filling | 1 | 60 | 2 | 8 | Tr | 1 |
| vanilla w/ creme filling | 1 | 50 | 2 | 7 | Tr | Tr |
| Shortbread cookie, plain | 1 | 45 | 2 | 6 | Tr | Tr |
| Shortbread w/fudge stripes | 1 | 65 | 3 | 9 | Tr | Tr |
| Sugar Cookie, regular | 1 | 65 | 3 | 8 | Tr | 1 |
| Sugar Cookie, reduced fat | 1 | 55 | 1 | 9 | Tr | 1 |
| Wafer, creme filled, | … | … | . | . | . | . |
| 2 ½" x 1" rectangles, | … | … | . | . | . | . |
| chocolate, creme filling | 3 | 140 | 7 | 18 | 1 | 1 |

| FOOD: (See Beverages & Fast Food Restaurants listed separately) | Serving Size | Calories | Fat (g) | Carb (g) | Fiber (g) | Protein (g) |
|---|---|---|---|---|---|---|
| sugarfree, w/ filling | 3 | 100 | 8 | 14 | Tr | 1 |
| vanilla, creme filling | 3 | 130 | 6 | 19 | Tr | 1 |
| Wafer, Vanilla, round, 1 ½" dia | 4 | 75 | 3 | 10 | Tr | 1 |
| Cooking Spray, nonstick | … | … | . | . | . | . |
| ¼ second spray | 1 spray | 0 | 0 | 0 | 0 | 0 |
| Corn | … | … | . | . | . | . |
| Sweet White, 5" cob, cooked | 1 ear | 83 | 1 | 19 | 2 | 3 |
| Sweet Yellow, on 5" cob, | … | … | . | . | . | . |
| fresh, cooked, 5" cob | 1 ear | 83 | 1 | 19 | 2 | 3 |
| frozen, cooked, 5" cob | 1 ear | 75 | 1 | 18 | 2 | 2 |
| frozen, cooked, kernels | ½ cup | 65 | Tr | 16 | 2 | 2 |
| canned, kernels, vacuum pack | ½ cup | 83 | 1 | 20 | 2 | 3 |
| canned, cream style kernels | ½ cup | 92 | 1 | 23 | 2 | 2 |
| Prep w/butter & herb sauce | ¾ cup | 180 | 4 | 30 | 2 | 5 |
| Corn Cake, butter flavor | 1 | 40 | Tr | 8 | 1 | 1 |
| (also see Rice Cake) | … | … | . | . | . | . |
| Corn Chips | … | … | . | . | . | . |
| Regular | 1 oz | 160 | 10 | 15 | 1 | 2 |
| Barbecue flavor | 1 oz | 170 | 10 | 17 | 1 | 2 |
| Ranch flavor | 1 oz | 150 | 7 | 20 | 1 | 2 |
| Reduced fat | 1 oz | 130 | 5 | 22 | 1 | 2 |
| Tortilla type | 1 oz | 140 | 7 | 17 | 1 | 2 |
| Doritos corn chips | 12 pc | 140 | 7 | 18 | 1 | 2 |
| Doritos nacho cheese | 12 pc | 140 | 7 | 18 | 1 | 2 |
| Doritos ranch | 12 pc | 140 | 7 | 18 | 1 | 2 |
| Doritos spicy nacho | 12 pc | 135 | 6 | 18 | 1 | 2 |
| Fritos corn chips, regular | 28 pc | 160 | 10 | 15 | 1 | 2 |
| Fritos BBQ corn chips | 28 pc | 160 | 9 | 16 | 1 | 2 |
| Fritos Chili cheese corn chips | 28 pc | 160 | 10 | 15 | 1 | 2 |
| Tostitos corn chips, round | 13 pc | 150 | 6 | 19 | 1 | 2 |
| Tostitos baked | 13 pc | 110 | 1 | 21 | 1 | 3 |
| Tostitos nacho | 6 pc | 150 | 6 | 19 | 1 | 2 |
| Tostitos restaurant style | 7 pc | 140 | 6 | 19 | 1 | 2 |
| Corn Grits (hominy) – see Grits | … | … | . | . | . | . |
| Corn Syrup | 1 Tbsp | 56 | 0 | 15 | 0 | 0 |
| Cornbread, 3" x 2" | 1 piece | 185 | 6 | 29 | 1 | 4 |
| Corned Beef, canned | 3 oz | 215 | 13 | 0 | 0 | 23 |
| Corned Beef Hash | 1 cup | 440 | 30 | 23 | 1 | 19 |
| Cornish Hen, roasted | 4 oz | 200 | 14 | 0 | 0 | 19 |
| Cornmeal, yellow, dry form | … | … | . | . | . | . |
| Whole grain | 1 cup | 440 | 4 | 94 | 9 | 10 |

| FOOD: (See Beverages & Fast Food Restaurants listed separately) | Serving Size | Calories | Fat (g) | Carb (g) | Fiber (g) | Protein (g) |
|---|---|---|---|---|---|---|
| Self rising | 1 cup | 490 | 2 | 103 | 10 | 12 |
| Cornstarch | 1 Tbsp | 30 | Tr | 7 | Tr | Tr |
| Cottage cheese – see Cheese | ... | ... | . | . | . | . |
| Crabcake | 1 | 150 | 4 | 12 | Tr | 9 |
| Cracker Jacks | ½ cup | 120 | 2 | 23 | 2 | 2 |
| **CRACKERS** | ... | ... | . | . | . | . |
| Butter flavor, round, 2" dia | 5 | 80 | 4 | 10 | Tr | 1 |
| Cheese crackers, 1" squares | 10 | 50 | 3 | 6 | Tr | 1 |
| Chicken in a Biskit | 12 | 160 | 8 | 17 | 1 | 2 |
| Club crackers | 4 | 70 | 3 | 9 | Tr | 1 |
| Club crackers, Keebler Club | 4 | 50 | 2 | 6 | Tr | Tr |
| Graham crackers, 2 ½" sq | 3 | 90 | 2 | 16 | Tr | 1 |
| Matzo, plain, 6" square | 1 | 120 | Tr | 25 | 1 | 3 |
| Melba toast, plain | 4 | 80 | 1 | 15 | Tr | 2 |
| Oat Thins | 9 | 70 | 3 | 10 | 1 | 2 |
| Oyster crackers | 25 | 65 | 1 | 11 | 1 | 1 |
| Ritz Bitz w/peanut butter | 13 | 150 | 8 | 17 | 1 | 4 |
| Ritz crackers, regular | 5 | 80 | 4 | 10 | Tr | 1 |
| Ritz crackers, reduced fat | 5 | 70 | 2 | 11 | Tr | 1 |
| Saltine crackers | 4 | 50 | 1 | 9 | Tr | 1 |
| Sandwich crackers, 1 ½" dia, | ... | ... | . | . | . | . |
| cheese crackers | 2 | 65 | 3 | 8 | Tr | 2 |
| peanut butter crackers | 2 | 65 | 3 | 8 | Tr | 2 |
| Snack crackers, round, 2" dia | 5 | 80 | 4 | 10 | Tr | 1 |
| Sociables | 7 | 80 | 4 | 9 | Tr | 1 |
| Town House crackers | 5 | 80 | 4 | 9 | Tr | 1 |
| Triscuit wafers | 7 | 140 | 5 | 21 | 1 | 3 |
| Vegetable crackers, thin squares | 7 | 80 | 4 | 10 | 1 | 2 |
| Wheat Thins | 9 | 60 | 2 | 10 | 1 | 1 |
| Wheatables | 8 | 70 | 3 | 10 | 1 | 1 |
| Whole wheat, thin squares | 8 | 75 | 4 | 10 | 1 | 2 |
| Zwieback | 2 | 70 | 2 | 12 | 1 | 2 |
| Cranberries | ... | . | . | . | . | . |
| Fresh, raw, unsweetened | ½ cup | 23 | Tr | 5 | 2 | Tr |
| Dried, sweetened | ¼ cup | 90 | Tr | 24 | 3 | Tr |
| Cranberry Relish | ¾ cup | 330 | 5 | 70 | 2 | 1 |
| Cranberry relish w/walnuts | ¾ cup | 365 | 6 | 75 | 3 | 3 |
| Cranberry Sauce, sweet, canned | 1 slice | 85 | Tr | 22 | 1 | Tr |
| Cream Cheese  - see Cheese | ... | ... | . | . | . | . |
| Cream of Tartar | 1 tsp | 8 | 0 | 2 | Tr | 0 |
| Cream of Wheat Cereal, as prep | 1 cup | 130 | Tr | 27 | 1 | 4 |

| FOOD:<br>(See Beverages & Fast Food Restaurants listed separately) | Serv-ing Size | Cal-ories | Fat (g) | Carb (g) | Fi-ber (g) | Pro-tein (g) |
|---|---|---|---|---|---|---|
| Cream, Whipped Topping | ... | ... | . | . | . | . |
|   Light | 1 cup | 700 | 75 | 7 | 0 | 5 |
|   Light | 1 Tbsp | 45 | 5 | Tr | 0 | Tr |
|   Heavy | 1 cup | 820 | 88 | 7 | 0 | 5 |
|   Heavy | 1 Tbsp | 50 | 6 | Tr | 0 | Tr |
|   Pressurized in can | 1 Tbsp | 8 | 1 | Tr | 0 | Tr |
| Creamer-see Beverages, Creamer | ... | ... | . | . | . | . |
| Croissant, butter flavor, 4" | 1 | 230 | 12 | 26 | 2 | 5 |
| Croissant w/Egg, Bacon, Cheese | 1 | 415 | 28 | 24 | 2 | 16 |
| Croissant w/Sausage | 1 | 440 | 32 | 29 | 2 | 13 |
| Croutons, seasoned | ½ cup | 92 | 3 | 13 | 1 | 2 |
| Cucumber | ... | ... | . | . | . | . |
|   Fresh, peeled, whole, 8" long | 1 | 35 | Tr | 7 | 2 | 2 |
|   Fresh, peeled, sliced | 1 cup | 14 | Tr | 3 | 1 | 1 |
|   Fresh, unpeeled, whole 8" long | 1 | 40 | Tr | 8 | 2 | 2 |
|   Fresh, unpeeled, sliced | 1 cup | 14 | Tr | 3 | 1 | 1 |
| Cucumber Salad, mayo dressing | ¾ cup | 120 | 10 | 9 | 2 | 2 |
| Cupcake, w/frosting, avg size,<br>  2 ¾" dia x 2 ¼" tall | ...<br>... | ...<br>... | .<br>. | .<br>. | .<br>. | .<br>. |
|   Banana | 1 | 190 | 6 | 32 | 1 | 1 |
|   Blueberry | 1 | 185 | 6 | 30 | 1 | 1 |
|   Chocolate | 1 | 195 | 6 | 32 | 1 | 2 |
|   Chocolate w/ crème filling | 1 | 190 | 7 | 31 | 1 | 1 |
|   Coconut w/ crème filling | 1 | 200 | 7 | 34 | 1 | 1 |
|   Strawberry | 1 | 185 | 6 | 30 | 1 | 1 |
|   Vanilla | 1 | 190 | 6 | 32 | Tr | 1 |
| Curry Powder | 1 tsp | 7 | Tr | 1 | Tr | Tr |
| Custard | ½ cup | 170 | 6 | 23 | Tr | 6 |
| Dandelion Greens, cooked | 1 cup | 35 | Tr | 7 | 3 | 2 |
| Danish Pastry | ... | ... | . | . | . | . |
|   Cheese, 4" dia | 1 | 265 | 15 | 26 | 1 | 6 |
|   Cinnamon & raisin, 4" dia | 1 | 260 | 12 | 33 | 2 | 5 |
|   Fruit filled, 4" dia | 1 | 260 | 12 | 34 | 1 | 4 |
|   Large, Cheese w/ fruit, 5" x 3" | 1 | 425 | 18 | 55 | 2 | 8 |
| Dates, pitted | ... | ... | . | . | . | . |
|   Whole | 5 dates | 115 | Tr | 30 | 3 | 1 |
|   Chopped | 1 cup | 490 | 1 | 130 | 13 | 4 |
| Dessert – see Ice Cream, Frozen<br>  Dessert, or specific listing | ...<br>... | ...<br>... | .<br>. | .<br>. | .<br>. | .<br>. |
| Dessert Filling - see specific | ... | ... | . | . | . | . |

| FOOD:<br>(See Beverages & Fast Food Restaurants listed separately) | Serv-ing Size | Cal-ories | Fat (g) | Carb (g) | Fi-ber (g) | Pro-tein (g) |
|---|---|---|---|---|---|---|
| listing | … | … | . | . | . | . |
| Dessert Topping – see Topping | … | … | . | . | . | . |
| Dill Weed, raw, sprigs | 5 | Tr | Tr | Tr | Tr | Tr |
| **Dip** | … | … | . | . | . | . |
| Avocado | 1 Tbsp | 30 | 2 | 2 | Tr | 1 |
| Bacon | 1 Tbsp | 30 | 2 | 2 | Tr | 1 |
| French Onion | 1 Tbsp | 25 | 2 | 1 | Tr | Tr |
| Ranch | 1 Tbsp | 30 | 2 | 2 | Tr | 1 |
| Sour Cream & Chives, regular | 1 Tbsp | 30 | 2 | 2 | Tr | 1 |
| Sour Cream & Chives, light | 1 Tbsp | 15 | Tr | 2 | Tr | 1 |
| **Doughnut** | … | … | . | . | . | . |
| Cake Doughnuts | … | … | . | . | . | . |
| Regular ring type, 3" dia | … | … | . | . | . | . |
| Plain | 1 | 200 | 11 | 23 | 1 | 2 |
| Powdered sugar | 1 | 240 | 11 | 33 | 1 | 3 |
| Chocolate frosting | 1 | 270 | 13 | 36 | 1 | 3 |
| Vanilla frosting & sprinkles | 1 | 280 | 13 | 39 | 1 | 3 |
| Holes or Munchkins | … | … | . | . | . | . |
| Cinnamon coated | 4 | 250 | 14 | 30 | 2 | 3 |
| Plain | 4 | 220 | 14 | 22 | 2 | 2 |
| Powdered sugar | 4 | 250 | 14 | 29 | 2 | 2 |
| Cruller glazed & frosted | … | … | . | . | . | . |
| w/chocolate | 1 | 280 | 15 | 35 | 1 | 2 |
| Yeast Doughnuts | … | … | . | … | . | . |
| Regular ring type, 3" dia | … | … | . | … | . | . |
| Glazed | 1 | 200 | 12 | 22 | 1 | 2 |
| Glazed & frosted w/vanilla | 1 | 250 | 12 | 33 | 1 | 3 |
| Glazed & frosted | … | … | . | . | . | . |
| w/chocolate & sprinkles | 1 | 270 | 12 | 36 | 1 | 3 |
| Holes or Munchkins | … | … | . | . | . | . |
| Glazed | 5 | 200 | 9 | 27 | 1 | 3 |
| Sugar coated | 6 | 220 | 12 | 26 | 1 | 4 |
| Filled doughnuts | … | … | . | . | . | . |
| Vanilla iced, crème filled | 1 | 360 | 19 | 41 | 2 | 5 |
| Powdered & strawberry | … | … | . | . | . | . |
| filled | 1 | 260 | 16 | 26 | 1 | 3 |
| Dressing – see Salad Dressing | … | … | . | . | . | . |
| Dried Fruit – see specific listings, and Trail Mix | …<br>… | …<br>… | .<br>. | .<br>. | .<br>. | .<br>. |
| Duck, roasted, ½ Duck, meat only | ½ duck | 445 | 25 | 0 | 0 | 52 |
| Dumpling, steamed, filled | … | … | . | . | . | . |

36

| FOOD: (See Beverages & Fast Food Restaurants listed separately) | Serv- ing Size | Cal- ories | Fat (g) | Carb (g) | Fi- ber (g) | Pro- tein (g) |
|---|---|---|---|---|---|---|
| w/meat, poultry, or seafood | 2 | 85 | 2 | 7 | 0.5 | 8 |
| Pot sticker dumpling | 2 | 144 | 6 | 15 | 1 | 5 |
| Éclair, 5" x 2" | 1 | 260 | 16 | 24 | 1 | 6 |
| **EGGs** | ... | ... | . | . | . | . |
| Raw Eggs | ... | ... | . | . | . | . |
| 1 medium whole egg | 1 | 65 | 4 | 1 | 0 | 5 |
| 1 large whole egg | 1 | 75 | 5 | 1 | 0 | 6 |
| 1 extra large whole egg | 1 | 85 | 6 | 1 | 0 | 7 |
| 1 yolk only, large | 1 | 60 | 5 | Tr | 0 | 3 |
| 1 white only, large | 1 | 15 | 0 | Tr | 0 | 4 |
| Prepared Eggs (1 Lg egg/svg) | ... | ... | . | . | . | . |
| deviled | 1 | 120 | 10 | 1 | 0 | 7 |
| hard boiled, whole | 1 | 75 | 5 | 1 | 0 | 6 |
| hard boiled, chopped | 1 cup | 210 | 14 | 2 | 0 | 17 |
| omelet, plain, milk added | 1 | 105 | 8 | 1 | 0 | 7 |
| pan fried in margarine | 1 | 92 | 7 | 1 | 0 | 6 |
| poached | 1 | 75 | 5 | 1 | 0 | 6 |
| scrambled w/margarine | ... | ... | . | . | . | . |
| & milk | 1 | 100 | 7 | 1 | 0 | 7 |
| Egg Substitute or imitation | ¼ cup | 35 | 1 | Tr | 0 | 6 |
| Eggplant | ... | ... | . | . | . | . |
| Cubed, cooked | 1 cup | 28 | Tr | 7 | 3 | 1 |
| Fried sticks | ½ cup | 240 | 12 | 28 | 3 | 4 |
| Eggplant Parmagiana | ½ cup | 265 | 16 | 26 | 3 | 6 |
| Eggroll | ... | ... | . | . | . | . |
| Chicken, Chun King entrée | 1 meal | 170 | 5 | 25 | 2 | 7 |
| Chicken, La Choy entrée | 1 meal | 170 | 5 | 25 | 2 | 7 |
| Pork, Chun King entrée | 1 meal | 170 | 6 | 23 | 2 | 6 |
| Pork eggroll, 4" long, 1 avg | 1 | 165 | 6 | 22 | 2 | 6 |
| Shrimp, Chun King entrée | 1 meal | 150 | 4 | 24 | 2 | 6 |
| Enchilada | ... | ... | . | . | . | . |
| Beef, Banquet entrée | 1meal | 380 | 12 | 54 | 1 | 15 |
| Beef, Patio entrée | 1 meal | 350 | 10 | 52 | 1 | 12 |
| Cheese, Banquet entrée | 1 meal | 340 | 6 | 56 | 1 | 15 |
| Chicken, Banquet entrée | 1 meal | 360 | 10 | 54 | 1 | 15 |
| Enchirito | ... | ... | . | . | . | . |
| Beef | 1 | 370 | 19 | 33 | 2 | 18 |
| Chicken | 1 | 350 | 16 | 32 | 2 | 21 |
| Steak | 1 | 350 | 16 | 31 | 2 | 22 |
| Endive, raw, chopped | 1 cup | 9 | Tr | 2 | 2 | 1 |
| Energy Bar, low carb | ... | ... | . | . | . | . |

| FOOD: (See Beverages & Fast Food Restaurants listed separately) | Serv- ing Size | Cal- ories | Fat (g) | Carb (g) | Fi- ber (g) | Pro- tein (g) |
|---|---|---|---|---|---|---|
| Atkins Advantage Chocolate | 1 bar | 220 | 11 | 25 | 11 | 17 |
| Atkins Advantage S'mores | 1 bar | 220 | 10 | 26 | 11 | 17 |
| English Muffin | ... | ... | . | . | . | . |
| Regular | 1 whole | 135 | 1 | 26 | 2 | 4 |
| Cinnamon raisin | 1 whole | 140 | 2 | 28 | 2 | 4 |
| English Muffin w/Egg, Cheese, | ... | ... | . | . | . | . |
| & Canadian Bacon | 1 | 290 | 13 | 27 | 2 | 17 |
| Equal sweetener | 1 pkt | 0 | 0 | Tr | 0 | 0 |
| Fajita, Chicken, Healthy Choice | 1 meal | 260 | 4 | 36 | 1 | 21 |
| Fettuccini Alfredo, w/ beef | 1 cup | 310 | 13 | 26 | 2 | 20 |
| Fig, fresh or dried, large | 2 | 98 | Tr | 25 | 5 | 1 |
| **FISH / SEAFOOD** | ... | ... | . | . | . | . |
| Abalone, fried | 3 oz | 160 | 6 | 9 | 1 | 17 |
| Anchovy, canned in oil | 5 | 42 | 2 | 0 | 0 | 6 |
| Bass | ... | ... | . | . | . | . |
| black, baked | 3 oz | 260 | 16 | 11 | 0 | 16 |
| striped, baked | 3 oz | 105 | 3 | 0 | 0 | 19 |
| Bluefish, baked | 3 oz | 135 | 5 | 0 | 0 | 22 |
| Catfish | ... | ... | . | . | . | . |
| baked or broiled | 3 oz | 130 | 5 | 0 | 0 | 20 |
| breaded, fried | 3 oz | 195 | 8 | 17 | 1 | 13 |
| Caviar, black or red | 2 Tbsp | 80 | 6 | 1 | 0 | 8 |
| Clams | ... | ... | . | . | . | . |
| breaded, fried | ¾ cup | 450 | 26 | 39 | Tr | 13 |
| canned, drained | 3 oz | 125 | 2 | 4 | 0 | 22 |
| canned, drained | 1 cup | 235 | 3 | 8 | 0 | 41 |
| raw | 3 oz | 63 | 1 | 2 | 0 | 11 |
| raw | 1 med | 11 | Tr | Tr | 0 | 2 |
| steamed | 3 oz | 125 | 2 | 4 | 0 | 22 |
| Cod, baked or broiled | 3 oz | 90 | 1 | 0 | 0 | 20 |
| Crab, Alaska king | ... | ... | . | . | . | . |
| steamed | 3 oz | 82 | 1 | 0 | 0 | 16 |
| steamed | 1 leg | 130 | 2 | 0 | 0 | 26 |
| Crab, blue | ... | ... | . | . | . | . |
| steamed | 3 oz | 88 | 2 | 0 | 0 | 17 |
| canned | 1 cup | 135 | 2 | 0 | 0 | 28 |
| Crab, imitation crab meat | 3 oz | 88 | 1 | 9 | 0 | 10 |
| Crab cake, w/egg, fried | 1 cake | 95 | 5 | 1 | 0 | 12 |
| Dolphinfish filet | 4 oz | 115 | 1 | 0 | 0 | 22 |
| Fish fillet, breaded, fried | 3 oz | 190 | 9 | 17 | 1 | 10 |
| Fish stick, breaded, fried, 3 x 1" | 2 sticks | 76 | 3 | 7 | Tr | 4 |

| FOOD: (See Beverages & Fast Food Restaurants listed separately) | Serv- ing Size | Cal- ories | Fat (g) | Carb (g) | Fi- ber (g) | Pro- tein (g) |
|---|---|---|---|---|---|---|
| Flounder | ... | ... | . | . | . | . |
| baked or broiled | 3 oz | 100 | 1 | 0 | 0 | 21 |
| breaded, fried fillet | 3 oz | 190 | 8 | 17 | 1 | 13 |
| Grouper, baked or broiled | 3 oz | 100 | 1 | 0 | 0 | 21 |
| Haddock | ... | ... | . | . | . | . |
| baked or broiled | 3 oz | 95 | 1 | 0 | 0 | 21 |
| breaded, fried fillet | 3 oz | 195 | 8 | 17 | 1 | 13 |
| Halibut | ... | ... | . | . | . | . |
| baked or broiled | 3 oz | 120 | 2 | 0 | 0 | 23 |
| breaded, fried fillet | 3 oz | 210 | 9 | 17 | 1 | 14 |
| Herring, pickled | 3 oz | 225 | 15 | 8 | 0 | 12 |
| Lobster, steamed | 3 oz | 85 | 1 | 1 | 0 | 17 |
| Lobster, imitation meat | 3 oz | 90 | 1 | 9 | 0 | 10 |
| Mackerel | ... | ... | . | . | . | . |
| baked or broiled | 3 oz | 225 | 15 | 0 | 0 | 20 |
| mackerel, jack, canned | 1 cup | 295 | 12 | 0 | 0 | 44 |
| Mahi Mahi filet | 4 oz | 115 | 1 | 0 | 0 | 22 |
| Monkfish, baked or broiled | 3 oz | 130 | 4 | 0 | 0 | 21 |
| Mussels, steamed | 3 oz | 145 | 4 | 6 | 0 | 20 |
| Orange roughy, baked or broiled | 3 oz | 75 | 1 | 0 | 0 | 16 |
| Oyster | ... | ... | . | . | . | . |
| raw meat | 1 cup | 170 | 6 | 10 | 0 | 17 |
| raw meat | 6 med | 55 | 2 | 3 | 0 | 6 |
| breaded, fried | 3 oz | 165 | 11 | 10 | 1 | 7 |
| Perch, baked or broiled | 3 oz | 105 | 2 | 0 | 0 | 20 |
| Pike, baked or broiled | 3 oz | 95 | 1 | 0 | 0 | 21 |
| Pollock, baked or broiled | 3 oz | 95 | 1 | 0 | 0 | 20 |
| Pompano, baked or broiled | 3 oz | 180 | 10 | 0 | 0 | 20 |
| Rockfish, baked or broiled | 3 oz | 105 | 2 | 0 | 0 | 20 |
| Salmon | ... | ... | . | . | . | . |
| baked or broiled | 3 oz | 185 | 9 | 0 | 0 | 23 |
| canned, pink | 3 oz | 118 | 5 | 0 | 0 | 17 |
| smoked, chinook | 3 oz | 100 | 4 | 0 | 0 | 16 |
| Sardine, canned in oil, drained | 3 oz | 175 | 10 | 0 | 0 | 21 |
| Scallop | ... | ... | . | . | . | . |
| breaded, fried | 6 large | 200 | 10 | 9 | Tr | 17 |
| steamed | 3 oz | 95 | 1 | 3 | 0 | 20 |
| Shark | ... | ... | . | . | . | . |
| Pacific shark, baked | 3 oz | 130 | 8 | 0 | 0 | 15 |
| thrasher, baked | 3 oz | 85 | 1 | 0 | 0 | 18 |
| Shrimp | ... | ... | . | . | . | . |

| FOOD:<br>(See Beverages & Fast Food<br>Restaurants listed separately) | Serv-ing Size | Cal-ories | Fat (g) | Carb (g) | Fi-ber (g) | Pro-tein (g) |
|---|---|---|---|---|---|---|
| breaded, fried | 2 large | 110 | 6 | 5 | Tr | 10 |
| breaded, fried | 3 oz | 205 | 10 | 10 | Tr | 18 |
| canned, drained | 3 oz | 100 | 2 | 1 | 0 | 20 |
| Snapper, baked or broiled | 3 oz | 110 | 2 | 0 | 0 | 22 |
| Sole | ... | ... | . | . | . | . |
|   baked or broiled | 3 oz | 100 | 1 | 0 | 0 | 21 |
|   breaded, fried fillet | 3 oz | 190 | 8 | 17 | 1 | 13 |
| Squid, fried | 3 oz | 150 | 6 | 7 | 0 | 15 |
| Swordfish | ... | ... | . | . | . | . |
|   baked | 3 oz | 130 | 4 | 0 | 0 | 22 |
|   broiled | 4 oz | 170 | 5 | 0 | 0 | 28 |
| Trout, baked or broiled | 3 oz | 145 | 6 | 0 | 0 | 21 |
| Tuna | ... | ... | . | . | . | . |
|   baked or broiled | 3 oz | 120 | 1 | 0 | 0 | 25 |
|   canned in oil, drained | 3 oz | 170 | 7 | 0 | 0 | 25 |
|   canned in water, chunk light | 3 oz | 100 | 1 | 0 | 0 | 22 |
|   canned in water, solid white | 3 oz | 110 | 3 | 0 | 0 | 20 |
|   tuna salad, oil packed, w/mayo | ½ cup | 190 | 10 | 9 | 0 | 16 |
|   tuna salad, water packed, w/ | ... | ... | . | . | . | . |
|     light mayo type dressing | ½ cup | 130 | 5 | 6 | 0 | 15 |
| Whiting, baked or broiled | 3 oz | 100 | 1 | 0 | 0 | 21 |
| Fish & Chips, Swanson entrée | 1 meal | 495 | 20 | 60 | 2 | 20 |
| Fish & Macaroni w/cheese | ... | ... | . | . | . | . |
|   Stouffers entrée | 1 meal | 460 | 20 | 47 | 2 | 22 |
| Fish Baked w/Lemon Pepper | ... | ... | . | . | . | . |
|   Healthy Choice entrée | 1 meal | 290 | 5 | 47 | 1 | 14 |
| Fish Florentine, Lean Cuisine | 1 meal | 240 | 9 | 13 | Tr | 27 |
| Fish Sandwich, 3 oz fried fish | ... | ... | . | . | . | . |
|   fillet with tarter sauce & cheese | 1 avg | 530 | 29 | 48 | Tr | 22 |
| Flank Steak – see Beef | ... | ... | . | . | . | . |
| Flour, unsifted | ... | ... | . | . | . | . |
|   All purpose flour, white | 1 cup | 455 | 1 | 95 | 3 | 13 |
|   Bread flour | 1 cup | 495 | 2 | 99 | 3 | 16 |
|   Buckwheat flour, whole groat | 1 cup | 400 | 4 | 85 | 12 | 15 |
|   Cake or pastry flour | 1 cup | 495 | 1 | 107 | 2 | 11 |
|   Carob flour | 1 cup | 230 | 1 | 92 | 41 | 5 |
|   Self-rising flour, white | 1 cup | 443 | 1 | 93 | 3 | 12 |
|   Whole wheat flour | 1 cup | 407 | 2 | 87 | 15 | 16 |
| Frankfurter – see Hot Dog | ... | ... | . | . | . | . |
| Freezer Pop – see Frozen Dessert | ... | ... | . | . | . | . |
| French Fries | ... | ... | . | . | . | . |

| FOOD:<br>(See Beverages & Fast Food Restaurants listed separately) | Serv-ing Size | Cal-ories | Fat (g) | Carb (g) | Fi-ber (g) | Pro-tein (g) |
|---|---|---|---|---|---|---|
| Frozen, heated, | … | … | . | . | . | . |
|    thin, shoestring strips, 3 oz | 20 fries | 130 | 4 | 22 | 2 | 2 |
|    thick or crinkle cuts, 4.5 oz | 20 fries | 195 | 6 | 33 | 3 | 3 |
|    Restaurant type, regular fries | 1 med | 350 | 15 | 48 | 5 | 5 |
|    Curly Cheddar Fries | 1 med | 460 | 24 | 54 | 5 | 6 |
|    Curly Fries | 1 med | 400 | 20 | 40 | 5 | 5 |
| French Toast | 2 slices | 250 | 8 | 38 | 1 | 8 |
| Fried Chicken – see Chicken | … | … | . | . | . | . |
| Fried Rice – see Rice | … | … | . | . | . | . |
| Frijoles | 1 cup | 225 | 8 | 29 | 2 | 11 |
| Frosting | … | … | . | . | . | . |
|    Chocolate | 1 Tbsp | 75 | 3 | 12 | Tr | Tr |
|    Vanilla | 1 Tbsp | 80 | 3 | 13 | Tr | Tr |
| **Frozen Dessert** | … | … | . | . | . | . |
|    (also see Ice Cream) | … | … | . | . | . | . |
|    Freezer Pop – (long tubes)_ | … | … | . | . | . | . |
|      Regular, fruit flavored, 1.5 oz | 1 | 25 | 0 | 6 | 0 | 0 |
|      Sugar free, fruit flav, 1.5 oz | 2 | 4 | 0 | 1 | 0 | 0 |
|    Frozen chocolate log cake | 1 slice | 280 | 9 | 43 | 1 | 5 |
|    Frozen chocolate round cake | 1 slice | 340 | 12 | 53 | 1 | 7 |
|    Fruit & Juice Bar, 2.5 oz | 1 | 65 | Tr | 16 | 0 | 1 |
|    Fudge Bar, 1.75 oz | 1 | 65 | Tr | 13 | Tr | 4 |
|    Ice Pop Bar, 2 oz | 1 | 45 | 0 | 11 | 0 | 0 |
|    Italian Ices | ½ cup | 65 | Tr | 16 | 0 | Tr |
|    Popsicle, 4 oz | 1 | 90 | 0 | 22 | 0 | 0 |
|    Vanilla Sandwich bar | 1 | 220 | 9 | 31 | 1 | 4 |
| Fruit  (see specific listings) | … | … | . | . | . | . |
|    Mixed, canned, w/light syrup | 1 cup | 150 | Tr | 39 | 2 | 2 |
|    Mixed, frozen, sweetened | 1 cup | 245 | Tr | 61 | 5 | 4 |
| Fruit Cocktail | … | … | . | . | . | . |
|    Canned in heavy syrup | 1 cup | 180 | Tr | 47 | 3 | 1 |
|    Canned in juice | 1 cup | 110 | Tr | 28 | 2 | 1 |
| Fruit Salad, mixed diced fruits | ¾ cup | 70 | 1 | 9 | 3 | 1 |
| Fudge | … | … | . | . | . | . |
|    Chocolate fudge, plain | 1 oz | 110 | 2 | 24 | Tr | 1 |
|    Chocolate fudge w/ nuts | 1 oz | 125 | 4 | 21 | Tr | 2 |
|    Vanilla fudge, plain | 1 oz | 105 | 1 | 23 | Tr | 1 |
|    Vanilla fudge, w/nuts | 1 oz | 120 | 4 | 22 | Tr | 1 |
| Funyuns  (snacks) | 13 | 140 | 7 | 18 | 1 | 2 |
| Garlic, raw | 1 clove | 4 | Tr | 1 | Tr | Tr |

| FOOD: (See Beverages & Fast Food Restaurants listed separately) | Serv-ing Size | Cal-ories | Fat (g) | Carb (g) | Fi-ber (g) | Pro-tein (g) |
|---|---|---|---|---|---|---|
| Garlic Powder or Salt | 1 tsp | 8 | Tr | 2 | Tr | Tr |
| Gelatin ( Jello ) | ... | ... | . | . | . | . |
| Banana, regular | ½ cup | 80 | 0 | 19 | 0 | 2 |
| Banana, sugar free | ½ cup | 10 | 0 | 1 | 0 | 1 |
| Cherry, regular | ½ cup | 75 | 0 | 18 | 0 | 2 |
| Cherry, sugar free | ½ cup | 10 | 0 | 1 | 0 | 1 |
| Orange, regular | ½ cup | 75 | 0 | 18 | 0 | 2 |
| Orange, sugar free | ½ cup | 10 | 0 | 1 | 0 | 1 |
| Raspberry, regular | ½ cup | 75 | 0 | 18 | 0 | 2 |
| Raspberry, sugar free | ½ cup | 10 | 0 | 1 | 0 | 1 |
| Strawberry , regular | ½ cup | 75 | 0 | 18 | 0 | 2 |
| Strawberry, sugar free | ½ cup | 10 | 0 | 1 | 0 | 1 |
| Gordita | ... | ... | . | . | . | . |
| Beef & cheese | 1 | 310 | 15 | 30 | 2 | 13 |
| Chicken & cheese | 1 | 290 | 13 | 29 | 2 | 15 |
| Steak & cheese | 1 | 290 | 13 | 28 | 2 | 16 |
| Granola Bar | ... | ... | . | . | . | . |
| Low fat, fruit variety,small bar | 1 bar | 90 | 1 | 19 | 2 | 3 |
| Plain granola bar | 1 bar | 135 | 6 | 18 | 2 | 3 |
| Chocolate chip | 1 bar | 150 | 6 | 22 | 1 | 3 |
| Chocolate chip & peanuts | 1 bar | 160 | 10 | 18 | 2 | 4 |
| Coconut | 1 bar | 140 | 6 | 20 | 1 | 3 |
| Raisin | 1 bar | 140 | 6 | 20 | 1 | 3 |
| Grapefruit, pink, red, or white | ... | ... | . | . | . | . |
| fresh, 3 ¾" dia | 1 | 80 | Tr | 18 | 3 | 2 |
| canned, in juice | 1 cup | 115 | Tr | 28 | 2 | 1 |
| canned, in light syrup | 1 cup | 150 | Tr | 39 | 1 | 1 |
| Grapes, seeded | ... | ... | . | . | . | . |
| Fresh, medium size, all types | 10 | 35 | Tr | 9 | 1 | Tr |
| Fresh, small or medium size | 1 cup | 115 | 1 | 28 | 2 | 1 |
| Gravy | ... | ... | . | . | . | . |
| Beef | ¼ cup | 40 | 2 | 4 | Tr | 2 |
| Chicken | ¼ cup | 32 | 1 | 3 | Tr | 2 |
| Country Sausage | ¼ cup | 60 | 4 | 4 | Tr | 2 |
| Mushroom | ¼ cup | 30 | 2 | 3 | Tr | 1 |
| Pork | ¼ cup | 38 | 2 | 3 | Tr | 2 |
| Turkey | ¼ cup | 31 | 1 | 3 | Tr | 2 |
| Grits, corn (hominy), as prep | 1 cup | 145 | Tr | 31 | 1 | 3 |
| Ground Beef – see Beef | ... | ... | . | . | . | . |
| Guava, raw, med size | 1 | 45 | Tr | 11 | 2 | 1 |
| Gum – see Chewing Gum | ... | ... | . | . | . | . |

| FOOD:<br>(See Beverages & Fast Food<br>Restaurants listed separately) | Serv-ing Size | Cal-ories | Fat (g) | Carb (g) | Fi-ber (g) | Pro-tein (g) |
|---|---|---|---|---|---|---|
| **HAM** (also see Pork) | ... | ... | . | . | . | . |
| Canned, regular, roasted | 3 oz | 155 | 9 | 2 | 0 | 15 |
| lean, roasted | 3 oz | 130 | 7 | 1 | 0 | 16 |
| Leg, roasted, lean & fat | 3 oz | 230 | 15 | 0 | 0 | 23 |
| lean only | 3 oz | 180 | 8 | 0 | 0 | 25 |
| Light cure, roasted, lean & fat | 3 oz | 205 | 14 | 0 | 0 | 18 |
| lean only | 3 oz | 135 | 5 | 0 | 0 | 21 |
| Lunch meat, 1/8" slices | ... | ... | . | . | . | . |
| regular | 2 slices | 150 | 5 | 3 | 0 | 21 |
| lean/ lowfat | 2 slices | 60 | 1 | 2 | 0 | 10 |
| baked | 2 slices | 100 | 2 | 2 | 0 | 16 |
| maple glazed | 2 slices | 120 | 2 | 6 | Tr | 18 |
| smoked | 2 slices | 110 | 2 | 4 | 0 | 18 |
| **Hamburger** & Cheeseburger | ... | ... | . | . | . | . |
| w/ catsup, mustard, lettuce, | ... | ... | . | . | . | . |
| & onion or pickle | ... | ... | . | . | . | . |
| 4 oz burger w/o cheese | 1 | 420 | 20 | 37 | 2 | 23 |
| 4 oz burger w/cheese | 1 | 520 | 30 | 38 | 2 | 28 |
| (also, see Beef- Ground | ... | ... | . | . | . | . |
| & Fast Food Restaurants) | ... | ... | . | . | . | . |
| Hamburger Helper | ... | ... | . | . | . | . |
| Beef Pasta | 1 cup | 270 | 10 | 26 | 2 | 20 |
| Beef Romanoff | 1 cup | 290 | 11 | 28 | 2 | 20 |
| Beef Taco | 1 cup | 310 | 13 | 31 | 2 | 21 |
| Beef Teriyaki | 1 cup | 290 | 10 | 34 | 2 | 18 |
| Cheesy Shells | 1 cup | 340 | 14 | 30 | 2 | 22 |
| Fettuccini Alfredo | 1 cup | 310 | 13 | 26 | 2 | 20 |
| Zesty Italian | 1 cup | 320 | 11 | 34 | 2 | 21 |
| Hash Browns – see Potatoes | ... | ... | . | . | . | . |
| Hearts of Palm, canned | 1 piece | 9 | Tr | 2 | 1 | 1 |
| Honey, 1 Tbsp | 1 Tbsp | 64 | 0 | 17 | Tr | Tr |
| Honey, 1 cup | 1 cup | 1030 | 0 | 279 | 1 | 1 |
| Honeydew Melon | ... | ... | . | . | . | . |
| Fresh, avg size 6 ½" melon, | ... | ... | . | . | . | . |
| cubed or diced | 1 cup | 60 | Tr | 16 | 1 | 1 |
| wedge, 1/8 of melon | 1 wedge | 55 | Tr | 15 | 1 | 1 |
| Horseradish, as prep | 1 tsp | 4 | Tr | 1 | Tr | Tr |
| HOT DOG (FRANKFURTER) | ... | ... | . | . | . | . |
| Beef or Pork | 1 | 145 | 13 | 1 | 0 | 5 |
| Chicken or Turkey | 1 | 115 | 10 | 2 | 0 | 6 |
| Lowfat, any meat | 1 | 75 | 5 | 3 | 0 | 5 |

43

| FOOD:<br>(See Beverages & Fast Food<br>Restaurants listed separately) | Serv-ing Size | Cal-ories | Fat (g) | Carb (g) | Fi-ber (g) | Pro-tein (g) |
|---|---|---|---|---|---|---|
| Fat free, any meat | 1 | 45 | 0 | 5 | 0 | 6 |
| Hot Dog  (meal as prep) | … | … | . | . | . | . |
| Hot Dog on Bun | … | … | . | . | . | . |
| w/ catsup & mustard | 1 avg | 245 | 15 | 19 | 1 | 10 |
| Hot Dog on Bun w/ chili | 1 avg | 295 | 13 | 31 | 1 | 14 |
| Corndog | 1 avg | 395 | 16 | 49 | 2 | 16 |
| Hummus, commercial | 1 Tbsp | 23 | 1 | 2 | 1 | 1 |
| Hush Puppies | 5 | 260 | 12 | 35 | 2 | 5 |
| **Ice Cream** | … | … | . | . | . | . |
| Chocolate | … | … | . | . | . | . |
| regular | ½ cup | 145 | 7 | 19 | 1 | 3 |
| reduced fat | ½ cup | 100 | 3 | 15 | 1 | 3 |
| Vanilla | … | … | . | . | . | . |
| regular | ½ cup | 135 | 7 | 16 | 0 | 2 |
| reduced fat | ½ cup | 90 | 3 | 15 | 0 | 3 |
| rich | ½ cup | 180 | 12 | 17 | 0 | 3 |
| soft ice cream in cone | 1 cone | 200 | 13 | 19 | 0 | 4 |
| soft in cone, chocolate dipped | 1 cone | 255 | 13 | 32 | 1 | 5 |
| Sherbet, Orange | ½ cup | 100 | 1 | 22 | 0 | 1 |
| Ice Cream Cone, 2 ½" cup only | 1 cup | 20 | 0 | 4 | 0 | 0 |
| Ice Cream Sandwich, vanilla | 1 | 220 | 9 | 31 | 1 | 4 |
| Ice Pop - See Frozen Dessert | … | … | . | . | . | . |
| Italian Ices | ½ cup | 65 | Tr | 16 | 0 | Tr |
| Italian Seasoning, dried spice | ½ tsp | 3 | 0 | Tr | Tr | Tr |
| Jalapeno – see Peppers | … | … | . | . | . | . |
| Jam | … | … | . | . | . | . |
| All flavors, regular | 1 Tbsp | 55 | Tr | 14 | Tr | Tr |
| All flavors, restaurant packet | 1 pkt | 39 | Tr | 10 | Tr | Tr |
| Jello – see Gelatin | … | … | . | . | . | . |
| Jelly | … | … | . | . | . | . |
| All flavors, regular | 1 Tbsp | 54 | Tr | 13 | Tr | Tr |
| All flavors, restaurant packet | 1 pkt | 40 | Tr | 10 | Tr | Tr |
| Kale | … | … | . | . | . | . |
| Fresh, raw | 1 cup | 17 | Tr | 4 | 2 | 1 |
| Fresh, chopped, cooked | 1 cup | 36 | Tr | 7 | 3 | 2 |
| Frozen, chopped, cooked | 1 cup | 39 | Tr | 7 | 3 | 3 |
| Ketchup, regular | 1 Tbsp | 18 | Tr | 4 | Tr | Tr |
| restaurant size packet | 1 pkt | 10 | Tr | 3 | Tr | Tr |
| Kiwi fruit, fresh, medium size | 1 | 45 | Tr | 11 | 3 | 1 |
| Knockwurst, beef, Boars Head | 1 wurst | 310 | 27 | 1 | Tr | 15 |

| FOOD:<br>(See Beverages & Fast Food Restaurants listed separately) | Serving Size | Cal-ories | Fat (g) | Carb (g) | Fi-ber (g) | Pro-tein (g) |
|---|---|---|---|---|---|---|
| Kohlrabi, cooked, slices | 1 cup | 48 | Tr | 11 | 2 | 3 |
| **Lamb** | ... | ... | . | . | . | . |
| (Braised, broiled, or roasted) | ... | ... | . | . | . | . |
| Arm chop, lean & fat | 3 oz | 295 | 20 | 0 | 0 | 26 |
| lean only | 3 oz | 235 | 12 | 0 | 0 | 30 |
| Leg of lamb, lean & fat | 3 oz | 220 | 14 | 0 | 0 | 22 |
| lean only | 3 oz | 160 | 7 | 0 | 0 | 24 |
| Loin chop, lean & fat | 3 oz | 270 | 20 | 0 | 0 | 21 |
| lean only | 3 oz | 185 | 8 | 0 | 0 | 25 |
| Rib roast, lean & fat | 3 oz | 305 | 25 | 0 | 0 | 18 |
| lean only | 3 oz | 195 | 11 | 0 | 0 | 22 |
| Lard, 1 cup | 1 cup | 1850 | 205 | 0 | 0 | 0 |
| Lard, 1 Tbsp | 1 Tbsp | 115 | 13 | 0 | 0 | 0 |
| Lasagna,  avg size 2 ½" x 4 " | ... | ... | . | . | . | . |
| w/ meat sauce | 1 | 360 | 12 | 52 | 2 | 18 |
| w/ zucchini | 1 | 330 | 2 | 58 | 3 | 20 |
| Leek, chopped, cooked | 1 cup | 32 | Tr | 8 | 1 | 1 |
| Lemon, fresh, 2 ¼" dia | 1 | 20 | Tr | 4 | 2 | 1 |
| Lentil, cooked | ½ cup | 115 | 1 | 20 | 8 | 9 |
| **Lettuce**,   fresh, raw | ... | ... | . | . | . | . |
| Bibb, Boston, Butterhead | ... | ... | . | . | . | . |
| whole head, 5" dia | 1 head | 21 | Tr | 4 | 2 | 2 |
| single leaf | 1 leaf | 1 | Tr | Tr | Tr | Tr |
| Iceberg, Crisphead | ... | . | Tr | . | . | . |
| whole head, 6" dia | 1 head | 65 | 1 | 11 | 8 | 5 |
| single leaf | 1 leaf | 1 | Tr | Tr | Tr | Tr |
| pieces, chopped or shredded | 1 cup | 8 | Tr | 1 | Tr | 1 |
| wedge slice, 1/6  of 6" head | 1 wedge | 11 | Tr | 2 | 1 | 1 |
| Loose leaf | ... | ... | . | . | . | . |
| single leaf | 1 leaf | 2 | Tr | Tr | Tr | Tr |
| pieces, shredded or chopped | 1 cup | 10 | Tr | 2 | 1 | 1 |
| Romaine or cos | ... | ... | . | . | . | . |
| innerleaf | 1 leaf | 1 | Tr | Tr | Tr | Tr |
| pieces, shredded | 1 cup | 8 | Tr | 1 | Tr | 1 |
| Lime, fresh, 2" dia | 1 | 20 | Tr | 5 | 2 | Tr |
| Linguini w/Clam sauce | ... | ... | . | . | . | . |
| Lean Cuisine entrée | 1 meal | 260 | 7 | 32 | 2 | 16 |
| Liver | ... | ... | . | . | . | . |
| Beef liver, fried | 3 oz | 185 | 7 | 7 | 0 | 23 |
| Chicken liver, simmered | 1 liver | 31 | 1 | Tr | 0 | 5 |
| Veal liver, braised | 3.5 oz | 165 | 7 | 0 | 0 | 22 |

| FOOD: (See Beverages & Fast Food Restaurants listed separately) | Serving Size | Calories | Fat (g) | Carb (g) | Fiber (g) | Protein (g) |
|---|---|---|---|---|---|---|
| Liverwurst, Boars Head | 2 oz | 170 | 15 | 1 | Tr | 8 |
| Lobster – see Fish / Seafood | … | … | . | . | . | . |
| Lo Mein w/Vegetables | 1 ½ cup | 230 | 4 | 40 | 3 | 8 |
| Lo Mein w/meat & vegetables | 1 ½ cup | 310 | 12 | 35 | 1 | 13 |
| **Lunch Meat** (thin 1/8" slices) | … | … | . | . | . | . |
| Beef or Pork, regular | 2 slices | 180 | 16 | 2 | 0 | 7 |
| Beef or Pork, lowfat | 2 slices | 110 | 9 | 2 | 0 | 6 |
| Beef or Pork, fat free | 2 slices | 60 | 1 | 3 | 0 | 8 |
| Chicken or Turkey , regular | 2 slices | 160 | 14 | 2 | 0 | 7 |
| Chicken or Turkey, lowfat | 2 slices | 100 | 8 | 2 | 0 | 6 |
| Chicken or Turkey, fat free | 2 slices | 60 | 1 | 3 | 0 | 8 |
| Ham, regular | 2 slices | 150 | 5 | 3 | 0 | 21 |
| Ham, lean/lowfat | 2 slices | 60 | 1 | 2 | 0 | 10 |
| (also see specific listings) | … | … | . | . | . | . |
| Macaroni, elbows | … | … | . | . | . | . |
| Dry, uncooked | 1 cup | 420 | 2 | 82 | 4 | 14 |
| Plain, cooked | 1 cup | 195 | 1 | 40 | 2 | 7 |
| Macaroni & Cheese | 1 cup | 300 | 10 | 40 | 3 | 10 |
| Mackerel – see Fish | … | … | . | . | . | . |
| Malt O Meal, as prep | 1 cup | 122 | Tr | 26 | 1 | 4 |
| Mandarin Oranges | … | … | . | . | . | . |
| Canned in light syrup | 1 cup | 154 | Tr | 41 | 2 | 1 |
| Mango | … | … | . | . | . | . |
| Fresh, peeled, 11 oz | 1 | 135 | 1 | 35 | 4 | 1 |
| Fresh, peeled, sliced | 1 cup | 105 | Tr | 28 | 3 | 1 |
| Manicotti, 3 cheese | 2 piece | 300 | 9 | 40 | 1 | 16 |
| Margarine | … | … | . | . | . | . |
| Regular, 4 sticks/Lb | 1 stick | 815 | 90 | 1 | 0 | 1 |
| Regular, hard or soft | 1 cup | 1625 | 185 | 1 | 0 | 2 |
| Regular, hard or soft | 1 Tbsp | 100 | 11 | Tr | 0 | Tr |
| Regular, hard or soft | 1 tsp | 34 | 4 | Tr | 0 | Tr |
| Reduced fat 50% | 1 cup | 1235 | 139 | 0 | 0 | 1 |
| Reduced fat 50% | 1 tsp | 25 | 3 | 0 | 0 | Tr |
| Fat free | 1 cup | 512 | Tr | 0 | 0 | Tr |
| Fat free | 1 Tbsp | 5 | 0 | 0 | 0 | 0 |
| Spread or blend type, regular | 1 Tbsp | 100 | 11 | Tr | 0 | Tr |
| Spread or blend w/ vegetable oil | … | … | . | . | . | . |
| & margarine, 33% reduced fat | 1 Tbsp | 60 | 7 | 0 | 0 | 0 |
| Marjoram, dried spice | 1 tsp | 2 | 0 | Tr | Tr | Tr |
| Marmalade | 1 Tbsp | 50 | Tr | 14 | Tr | Tr |

| FOOD: (See Beverages & Fast Food Restaurants listed separately) | Serv-ing Size | Cal-ories | Fat (g) | Carb (g) | Fi-ber (g) | Pro-tein (g) |
|---|---|---|---|---|---|---|
| Marshmallow | … | … | . | . | . | . |
|   Miniature size | 1 cup | 160 | Tr | 41 | Tr | Tr |
|   Regular size | 2 piece | 46 | Tr | 12 | Tr | Tr |
|   Regular or Large size | 1 oz | 90 | Tr | 23 | Tr | Tr |
| Marshmallow Topping | 1 Tbsp | 50 | Tr | 12 | Tr | Tr |
| Mayonnaise | … | … | . | . | . | . |
|   Regular | 1 Tbsp | 100 | 11 | Tr | 0 | Tr |
|   Light / reduced calorie | 1 Tbsp | 50 | 5 | 1 | 0 | Tr |
|   Fat free | 1 Tbsp | 10 | 0 | 2 | 0 | Tr |
| Meat – see specific listings | … | … | . | . | . | . |
| Meat Tenderizer | ¼ tsp | 0 | 0 | 0 | 0 | 0 |
| Meatless Burger | … | … | . | . | . | . |
|   Single patty, broiled | 1 patty | 100 | 1 | 9 | 4 | 15 |
|   Cooked, crumbled | 1 cup | 230 | 13 | 7 | 5 | 22 |
| Meatloaf | … | … | . | . | . | . |
|   Banquet entrée | 1 meal | 280 | 16 | 22 | 1 | 13 |
|   Healthy Choice entrée | 1 meal | 320 | 5 | 52 | 1 | 15 |
|   Lean Cuisine entrée | 1 meal | 260 | 7 | 28 | 1 | 20 |
|   Meatloaf & cheese sandwich | 1 | 350 | 13 | 41 | 2 | 18 |
| Minestrone – see Soup | … | … | . | . | . | . |
| Molasses, blackstrap, 1 Tbsp | 1 Tbsp | 47 | 0 | 12 | 0 | 0 |
|   Molasses, blackstrap, 1 cup | 1 cup | 771 | 0 | 199 | 0 | 0 |
| Mortadella | 1 slice | 50 | 4 | Tr | 0 | 2 |
| **Muffin** | … | … | . | . | . | . |
|   Avg size muffin, 2 ½" dia | … | … | . | . | . | . |
|     Apple muffin | 1 | 160 | 4 | 28 | 2 | 3 |
|     Banana muffin | 1 | 165 | 4 | 29 | 2 | 3 |
|     Blueberry muffin | 1 | 160 | 4 | 28 | 2 | 3 |
|     Bran w/ raisins | 1 | 175 | 5 | 36 | 4 | 4 |
|     Chocolate Chip muffin | 1 | 180 | 5 | 37 | 2 | 3 |
|     Corn muffin | 1 | 175 | 5 | 29 | 2 | 3 |
|   Extra large muffin, 4" dia | … | … | . | . | . | . |
|     Banana nut muffin | 1 | 420 | 11 | 75 | 8 | 7 |
|     Bran w/raisins | 1 | 425 | 11 | 76 | 8 | 8 |
|   (also see English Muffin) | … | … | . | . | . | . |
| Mulberries | ½ cup | 30 | Tr | 7 | 3 | Tr |
| Mushroom | … | … | . | . | . | . |
|   Regular Mushrooms | … | … | . | . | . | . |
|     Fresh, raw, slices | 1 cup | 18 | Tr | 3 | 1 | 2 |
|     Fresh, sliced, cooked | 1 cup | 42 | Tr | 8 | 3 | 3 |
|     Canned, stems & pieces, | … | … | . | . | . | . |

| FOOD:  (See Beverages & Fast Food Restaurants listed separately) | Serv- ing Size | Cal- ories | Fat (g) | Carb (g) | Fi- ber (g) | Pro- tein (g) |
|---|---|---|---|---|---|---|
| cooked | 1 cup | 37 | Tr | 8 | 4 | 3 |
| Shiitake Mushrooms | ... | ... | . | . | . | . |
| Dried, cut pieces, cooked | 1 cup | 80 | Tr | 20 | 3 | 2 |
| Dried, whole, cooked | 1 whole | 11 | Tr | 3 | Tr | Tr |
| Mussels – see Fish/Seafood | ... | ... | . | . | . | . |
| Mustard, yellow | ... | ... | . | . | . | . |
| Regular | 1 tsp | 4 | Tr | Tr | Tr | Tr |
| Hot or Honey flavored | 1 tsp | 8 | Tr | 2 | Tr | Tr |
| Powder | 1 tsp | 10 | Tr | 2 | Tr | Tr |
| Mustard Greens, chopped, cooked | 1 cup | 21 | Tr | 3 | 2 | 3 |

| FOOD:  (See Beverages & Fast Food Restaurants listed separately) | Serv- ing Size | Cal- ories | Fat (g) | Carb (g) | Fi- ber (g) | Pro- tein (g) |
|---|---|---|---|---|---|---|
| Nachos w/ Cheese sauce | 7 pc | 345 | 19 | 36 | 3 | 9 |
| Nectarine, fresh, med, 2 ½" dia | 1 | 67 | 1 | 16 | 2 | 1 |
| Noodles   (egg noodles) | ... | ... | . | . | . | . |
| Dry, uncooked | 1 cup | 420 | 2 | 82 | 4 | 14 |
| Plain, cooked | 1 cup | 195 | 1 | 40 | 2 | 7 |
| Chow Mein noodles, | ... | ... | . | . | . | . |
| dry crunchy | 1 cup | 235 | 14 | 26 | 2 | 4 |
| Spinach noodles, cooked | 1 cup | 210 | 3 | 39 | 4 | 8 |
| Noodles Alfredo | ¾ cup | 250 | 7 | 39 | 2 | 10 |
| Noodles Stroganoff | ¾ cup | 220 | 4 | 37 | 2 | 9 |
| Nut Pastry Filling | 1 Tbsp | 65 | 2 | 13 | 1 | 2 |
| **Nuts** | ... | ... | . | . | . | . |
| Almonds | ... | ... | . | . | . | . |
| sliced almonds | 1 cup | 550 | 48 | 19 | 11 | 20 |
| whole almonds, about 24 | 1 oz | 165 | 14 | 6 | 3 | 6 |
| Brazil nuts, shelled, 6 to 8 nuts | 1 oz | 185 | 19 | 4 | 2 | 4 |
| Cashews | ... | ... | . | . | . | . |
| dry roasted, about 20 | 1 oz | 160 | 13 | 9 | 1 | 4 |
| oil roasted, about 18 | 1 oz | 165 | 14 | 8 | 1 | 5 |
| Chestnuts, roasted, shelled | 1 cup | 350 | 3 | 76 | 7 | 5 |
| Coconut | ... | ... | . | . | . | . |
| fresh, shredded | 1 cup | 285 | 27 | 12 | 7 | 3 |
| dried, sweetened flakes | 1 cup | 465 | 33 | 44 | 4 | 3 |

| FOOD:  (See Beverages & Fast Food  Restaurants listed separately) | Serv- ing Size | Cal- ories | Fat (g) | Carb (g) | Fi- ber (g) | Pro- tein (g) |
|---|---|---|---|---|---|---|
| Hazelnuts, chopped, ¼ cup | 1 oz | 180 | 17 | 5 | 3 | 4 |
| Macadamia, dry roasted, 11 nuts | 1 oz | 205 | 22 | 4 | 2 | 2 |
| Mixed Nuts w/ peanuts | … | … | . | . | . | . |
| dry roasted, about 20 nuts | 1 oz | 168 | 15 | 7 | 3 | 5 |
| oil roasted, about 20 nuts | 1 oz | 175 | 16 | 6 | 3 | 5 |
| Peanuts | … | … | . | . | . | . |
| dry roasted, unsalted | 1 cup | 855 | 73 | 31 | 12 | 35 |
| dry roasted, unsalted, about 28 | 1 oz | 165 | 14 | 6 | 2 | 7 |
| dry roasted, salted, about 28 | 1 oz | 165 | 14 | 6 | 2 | 7 |
| honey roasted, about 28 | 1 oz | 165 | 13 | 7 | 2 | 7 |
| oil roasted, salted, about 26 | 1 oz | 170 | 15 | 5 | 3 | 7 |
| Pecans, 10 whole or 20 halves | 1 oz | 195 | 20 | 4 | 3 | 3 |
| Pine nuts, shelled | 1 oz | 160 | 14 | 4 | 1 | 7 |
| Pistachio nuts, dry roasted, | … | … | . | . | . | . |
| shelled, about 47 | 1 oz | 160 | 13 | 8 | 3 | 6 |
| Walnuts, English | … | … | . | . | . | . |
| chopped | 1 cup | 785 | 78 | 16 | 8 | 18 |
| whole, 7 walnuts | 1 oz | 185 | 18 | 4 | 2 | 4 |
| Oat Bran | … | … | . | . | . | . |
| Uncooked | 1 cup | 230 | 7 | 62 | 15 | 16 |
| Cooked | 1 cup | 88 | 2 | 25 | 6 | 7 |
| Oatmeal, as prep | … | … | . | . | . | . |
| Plain, sweetened | ½ cup | 75 | 1 | 13 | 2 | 3 |
| Fruit flavored oatmeal | 1 pkt | 135 | 2 | 26 | 2 | 3 |
| Maple & brown sugar oatmeal | 1 pkt | 130 | 1 | 27 | 6 | 3 |
| Oats, dry, 100% rolled oats | ½ cup | 150 | 3 | 26 | 4 | 5 |
| OIL  (for cooking & salads) | … | … | . | . | . | . |
| Cooking spray, ¼ second spray | 1 spray | 0 | 0 | 0 | 0 | 0 |
| Canola oil | 1 cup | 1925 | 218 | 0 | 0 | 0 |
| Canola oil | Tbsp | 120 | 14 | 0 | 0 | 0 |
| Corn oil | 1 cup | 1925 | 218 | 0 | 0 | 0 |
| Corn oil | Tbsp | 120 | 14 | 0 | 0 | 0 |
| Cottonseed/soybean oil blend | 1 cup | 1925 | 218 | 0 | 0 | 0 |
| Cottonseed/soybean oil blend | 1 Tbsp | 120 | 14 | 0 | 0 | 0 |
| Olive oil | 1 cup | 1905 | 216 | 0 | 0 | 0 |
| Olive oil | 1 Tbsp | 119 | 14 | 0 | 0 | 0 |
| Peanut oil | 1 cup | 1905 | 216 | 0 | 0 | 0 |
| Peanut oil | 1 Tbsp | 119 | 14 | 0 | 0 | 0 |
| Safflower oil | 1 cup | 1925 | 218 | 0 | 0 | 0 |
| Safflower oil | 1 Tbsp | 120 | 14 | 0 | 0 | 0 |
| Sesame oil | 1 cup | 1925 | 218 | 0 | 0 | 0 |

| FOOD: (See Beverages & Fast Food Restaurants listed separately) | Serv- ing Size | Cal- ories | Fat (g) | Carb (g) | Fi- ber (g) | Pro- tein (g) |
|---|---|---|---|---|---|---|
| Sesame oil | 1 Tbsp | 120 | 14 | 0 | 0 | 0 |
| Soybean oil | 1 cup | 1925 | 218 | 0 | 0 | 0 |
| Soybean oil | 1 Tbsp | 120 | 14 | 0 | 0 | 0 |
| Sunflower oil | 1 cup | 1925 | 218 | 0 | 0 | 0 |
| Sunflower oil | 1 Tbsp | 120 | 14 | 0 | 0 | 0 |
| Vegetable oil | 1 cup | 1925 | 218 | 0 | 0 | 0 |
| Vegetable oil | 1 Tbsp | 120 | 14 | 0 | 0 | 0 |
| Okra | ... | ... | . | . | . | . |
| Fresh, sliced, cooked | 1 cup | 51 | Tr | 12 | 4 | 3 |
| Frozen, slices, cooked | 1 cup | 52 | 1 | 11 | 5 | 4 |
| Whole, 3" pods, cooked | 8 pods | 30 | Tr | 7 | 2 | 2 |
| Fried, breaded | ½ cup | 165 | 10 | 17 | 4 | 3 |
| Olive | ... | ... | . | . | . | . |
| Pickled, green, medium size | 5 | 20 | 2 | Tr | Tr | Tr |
| Ripe, black, large size | 5 | 25 | 2 | 1 | Tr | Tr |
| Olive Loaf | 2 oz | 130 | 12 | 1 | Tr | 6 |
| Onion | ... | ... | . | . | . | . |
| Round yellow or white onion | ... | ... | . | . | . | . |
| Fresh, raw, whole, 2 ½" dia | 1 whole | 42 | Tr | 9 | 2 | 1 |
| Fresh, chopped | 1 cup | 61 | Tr | 14 | 3 | 2 |
| Fresh, sliced, 1/8" thick | 1 slice | 5 | Tr | 1 | Tr | Tr |
| Cooked, whole, 2 ½" dia | 1 whole | 41 | Tr | 10 | 1 | 1 |
| Cooked, sliced or chopped | 1 cup | 92 | Tr | 21 | 3 | 3 |
| Sprigs w/green tops & bulbs | ... | ... | . | . | . | . |
| Whole w/top, raw, chopped | 1 whole | 8 | Tr | 1 | Tr | 1 |
| Bulbs only, chopped | 1 cup | 32 | Tr | 7 | 3 | 2 |
| Onion Flakes, dried | 1 Tbsp | 16 | Tr | 4 | Tr | Tr |
| Onion Powder or Salt | 1 tsp | 7 | Tr | 2 | Tr | Tr |
| Onion Rings | ... | ... | . | . | . | . |
| Breaded, fried | 5 rings | 125 | 7 | 13 | 1 | 2 |
| Orange | ... | ... | . | . | . | . |
| Fresh, medium size, 3" dia | 1 | 70 | Tr | 15 | 3 | 1 |
| Fresh, sections | 1 cup | 85 | Tr | 20 | 4 | 2 |
| Oregano, ground | 1 tsp | 5 | Tr | 1 | Tr | Tr |
| Pam, non-stick cooking spray | ... | ... | . | . | . | . |
| ¼ second spray | 1 spray | 0 | 0 | 0 | 0 | 0 |
| Pancake, 4" dia | ... | ... | . | . | | . |
| Regular, toaster type | 1 | 82 | 1 | 16 | 1 | 2 |
| Lowfat, toaster type | 1 | 70 | Tr | 17 | 1 | 2 |
| Regular, from mix or scratch | 1 | 90 | 2 | 17 | 1 | 2 |
| Blueberry, mix or toaster type | 1 | 85 | 1 | 15 | 1 | 2 |

| FOOD:<br>(See Beverages & Fast Food<br>Restaurants listed separately) | Serv-ing Size | Cal-ories | Fat (g) | Carb (g) | Fi-ber (g) | Pro-tein (g) |
|---|---|---|---|---|---|---|
| Pancake Syrup - see Syrup | ... | ... | . | . | . | . |
| Papaya | ... | ... | . | . | . | . |
| Fresh, peeled, 5" long x 3" dia | 1 | 120 | Tr | 30 | 6 | 2 |
| Fresh, peeled, cubed | 1 cup | 55 | Tr | 14 | 3 | 1 |
| Paprika, dried powder | 1 tsp | 6 | Tr | 1 | Tr | Tr |
| Parsley | ... | ... | . | . | . | . |
| Fresh, raw, chopped | 10 | 4 | Tr | 1 | Tr | Tr |
| Dried parsley bits | 1 Tbsp | 4 | Tr | 1 | Tr | Tr |
| Parsnip, sliced, cooked | 1 cup | 125 | Tr | 30 | 6 | 2 |
| Passion Fruit, raw, avg size | 1 | 17 | Tr | 4 | Tr | Tr |
| Pasta | ... | ... | . | . | . | . |
| Plain, cooked | 1 cup | 195 | 1 | 40 | 2 | 7 |
| W/cheese & tomato sauce | 1 cup | 250 | 6 | 41 | 3 | 7 |
| W/meatballs in tomato sauce | 1 cup | 260 | 10 | 31 | 3 | 11 |
| W/shrimp & herb sauce | 1 cup | 295 | 10 | 40 | 3 | 10 |
| W/tomato sauce | 1 cup | 240 | 5 | 41 | 3 | 7 |
| Pasta Roni | ... | ... | . | . | . | . |
| Pasta w/broccoli | 1 cup | 240 | 4 | 37 | 3 | 7 |
| Pasta w/broccoli & chicken | 1 cup | 260 | 5 | 37 | 3 | 8 |
| Pasta Alfredo Primavera | 1 cup | 280 | 7 | 44 | 3 | 11 |
| Pasta, Angel Hair | ... | ... | . | . | . | . |
| Prep w/herb sauce | 1 cup | 280 | 9 | 42 | 3 | 7 |
| Weight Watchers entrée | 1 meal | 170 | 2 | 29 | 2 | 8 |
| Pasta, Bowtie w/tomato sauce | 1 cup | 240 | 5 | 41 | 3 | 7 |
| Pasta Marsala | 1 cup | 280 | 9 | 36 | 3 | 13 |
| Pasta Salad w/dressing | 1 cup | 250 | 10 | 32 | 2 | 5 |
| Pastrami | ... | ... | . | . | . | . |
| Regular | 2 oz | 90 | 4 | 2 | Tr | 12 |
| Turkey | 2 oz | 60 | 1 | 1 | Tr | 13 |
| Pastry - see Danish Pastry &<br>   specific listings | ...<br>... | ...<br>... | .<br>. | .<br>. | .<br>. | .<br>. |
| Pastry Filling -see specific listing | ... | ... | . | . | . | . |
| Peach | ... | ... | . | . | . | . |
| Fresh, whole, med, 2 ½" dia | 1 | 42 | Tr | 11 | 2 | 1 |
| Fresh, sliced | 1 cup | 76 | Tr | 19 | 3 | 1 |
| Canned, in heavy syrup | 1 cup | 195 | Tr | 52 | 3 | 1 |
| Canned, in light syrup | 1 cup | 150 | Tr | 39 | 2 | 1 |
| Canned, in juice | 1 cup | 115 | Tr | 28 | 3 | 2 |
| Dried, halves, | 3 halves | 93 | Tr | 24 | 3 | 1 |
| Frozen, sweetened slices, thawed | 1 cup | 235 | Tr | 60 | 5 | 2 |

| FOOD: (See Beverages & Fast Food Restaurants listed separately) | Serving Size | Calories | Fat (g) | Carb (g) | Fiber (g) | Protein (g) |
|---|---|---|---|---|---|---|
| Peanut - see Nuts | ... | ... | . | . | . | . |
| Peanut Butter | ... | ... | . | . | . | . |
|   Regular, smooth | 1 Tbsp | 95 | 8 | 3 | 1 | 4 |
|   Regular, chunky | 1 Tbsp | 95 | 8 | 3 | 1 | 4 |
|   Reduced fat, smooth | 1 Tbsp | 90 | 6 | 6 | 1 | 5 |
| Pear | ... | ... | . | . | . | . |
|   Fresh, 2 ½" dia | 1 | 50 | Tr | 13 | 4 | 1 |
|   Fresh, 3 ¼" dia | 1 | 116 | 1 | 29 | 9 | 1 |
|   Canned, in heavy syrup | 1 cup | 197 | Tr | 51 | 4 | 1 |
|   Canned, in juice | 1 cup | 125 | Tr | 32 | 4 | 1 |
| Peas   (cooked w/o fats) | ... | ... | . | . | . | . |
|   Black eyed peas | ½ cup | 105 | Tr | 26 | 8 | 4 |
|   Chickpeas | ½ cup | 140 | 2 | 25 | 6 | 7 |
|   Green peas | ½ cup | 60 | Tr | 11 | 4 | 4 |
|   Lentils | ½ cup | 115 | 1 | 20 | 8 | 9 |
|   Navy peas | ½ cup | 125 | 1 | 24 | 6 | 8 |
|   Pea Pods | ½ cup | 40 | Tr | 7 | 2 | 3 |
|   Split peas | ½ cup | 115 | 1 | 20 | 8 | 8 |
|   Sweet peas | ½ cup | 60 | Tr | 11 | 4 | 4 |
| Peas and Carrots | ½ cup | 40 | Tr | 8 | 3 | 3 |
| Pecan Pastry Filling | 1 Tbsp | 65 | 2 | 13 | 1 | 2 |
| Pecans, 10 whole or 20 halves | 1 oz | 195 | 20 | 4 | 3 | 3 |
| Pepper, dried powder or granules | ... | ... | . | . | . | . |
|   Black | 1 tsp | 5 | Tr | 1 | Tr | Tr |
|   Cayenne or red | 1 tsp | 7 | Tr | 1 | Tr | Tr |
|   White | 1 tsp | 5 | Tr | 1 | Tr | Tr |
| Pepper Steak | ... | ... | . | . | . | . |
|   Stouffer's entree | 1 meal | 330 | 9 | 45 | 1 | 17 |
|   Le Menu entree | 1 meal | 354 | 13 | 35 | 1 | 26 |
| Pepperoni, 14 thin slices/oz | 1 oz | 130 | 12 | 0 | 0 | 6 |
| Peppers | ... | ... | . | . | . | . |
|   Chili Peppers, hot, raw | ... | ... | . | . | . | . |
|     red or green | 1 whole | 18 | Tr | 4 | 1 | 1 |
|   Green, sweet, raw | ... | ... | . | . | . | . |
|     whole, 3" x 2 ¼" | 1 whole | 32 | Tr | 8 | 2 | 1 |
|     ring, ¼" thick | 1 ring | 3 | Tr | 1 | Tr | Tr |
|     chopped | 1 cup | 40 | Tr | 10 | 3 | 1 |
|   Jalapeno peppers, sliced | ¼ cup | 7 | Tr | 1 | Tr | Tr |
|   Red, sweet, raw | ... | ... | . | . | . | . |
|     whole, 3" x 2 ¼" | 1 whole | 32 | Tr | 8 | 2 | 1 |
|     ring, ¼" thick | 1 ring | 3 | Tr | 1 | Tr | Tr |

| FOOD: (See Beverages & Fast Food Restaurants listed separately) | Serving Size | Calories | Fat (g) | Carb (g) | Fiber (g) | Protein (g) |
|---|---|---|---|---|---|---|
| chopped | 1 cup | 40 | Tr | 10 | 3 | 1 |
| Red or Green, sweet, cooked | ... | ... | . | . | . | . |
| chopped | 1 cup | 38 | Tr | 9 | 2 | 1 |
| Peppers, Stuffed, Stouffers | 1 cup | 200 | 5 | 27 | 3 | 11 |
| Persimmon, raw, medium size | 1 | 32 | Tr | 8 | 2 | Tr |
| Pickle | ... | ... | . | . | . | . |
| Bread & Butter slices, 1 ½" dia | 6 slices | 36 | Tr | 8 | 1 | Tr |
| Dill, whole, 3 ¾" long | 1 | 12 | Tr | 3 | 1 | Tr |
| Sweet Gherkin, 2 ½" long | 1 | 20 | Tr | 5 | Tr | Tr |
| Pickle Relish | 1 Tbsp | 20 | Tr | 5 | Tr | Tr |
| Pie  (1/8 of 9" pie unless noted) | ... | ... | . | . | . | . |
| Apple pie, 2 crust | 1 slice | 420 | 19 | 59 | 4 | 4 |
| Blueberry pie, 2 crust | 1 slice | 360 | 17 | 49 | 4 | 4 |
| Boston Cream Pie, 1 crust | 1 slice | 230 | 8 | 39 | 1 | 2 |
| Cherry pie, 2 crust | 1 slice | 485 | 22 | 69 | 4 | 5 |
| Cherry, fried pie, 4" x 2" | 1 slice | 405 | 21 | 55 | 3 | 4 |
| Chocolate chip pie, 1 crust | 1 slice | 590 | 34 | 57 | 3 | 6 |
| Chocolate Cream pie, 1 crust | 1 slice | 405 | 22 | 45 | 3 | 4 |
| Coconut Custard pie, 1 crust | 1 slice | 305 | 15 | 36 | 2 | 7 |
| Lemon Meringue pie, 1 crust | 1 slice | 360 | 16 | 50 | 1 | 5 |
| Peach pie, 2 crust | 1 slice | 410 | 19 | 58 | 3 | 4 |
| Pecan pie, 1 crust | 1 slice | 505 | 27 | 64 | 2 | 6 |
| Pumpkin pie, 1 crust | 1 slice | 320 | 14 | 41 | 3 | 7 |
| Strawberry pie, 2 crust | 1 slice | 360 | 16 | 50 | 2 | 5 |
| Pie Crust, 9" dia | ... | ... | . | . | . | . |
| Regular from recipe or frozen | 1 crust | 800 | 50 | 75 | 2 | 9 |
| Graham cracker crust | 1 crust | 950 | 51 | 110 | 3 | 9 |
| Reduced fat crust | 1 crust | 605 | 30 | 74 | 2 | 8 |
| Pilaf - see Rice Pilaf | ... | ... | . | . | . | . |
| Pimiento | 1 oz | 10 | Tr | 2 | Tr | Tr |
| Pineapple | ... | ... | . | . | . | . |
| Fresh, diced or sliced | 1 cup | 76 | 1 | 19 | 2 | 1 |
| Canned, in heavy syrup, | ... | ... | . | . | . | . |
| chunks or crushed | 1 cup | 198 | Tr | 51 | 2 | 1 |
| slices, 3" dia | 1 slice | 38 | Tr | 10 | Tr | Tr |
| Canned, in juice, | ... | ... | . | . | . | . |
| chunks or crushed | 1 cup | 150 | Tr | 39 | 2 | 1 |
| slices, 3" dia | 1 slice | 28 | Tr | 7 | 1 | Tr |
| PIZZA  (Listings for an avg size slice, 1/8 of 12" pizza) | ... | ... | . | . | . | . |
| Thin & Crispy Pizza | ... | ... | . | . | . | . |

| FOOD: (See Beverages & Fast Food Restaurants listed separately) | Serving Size | Calories | Fat (g) | Carb (g) | Fiber (g) | Protein (g) |
|---|---|---|---|---|---|---|
| Cheese | 1 slice | 140 | 3 | 21 | 1 | 8 |
| Pepperoni & Cheese | 1 slice | 180 | 7 | 20 | 1 | 10 |
| One Meat w/ Vegetables | 1 slice | 185 | 5 | 21 | 2 | 13 |
| Three Meat w/ Vegetables | 1 slice | 210 | 9 | 21 | 2 | 12 |
| Thick & Chewy or Pan Pizza | ... | ... | . | . | . | . |
| Cheese | 1 slice | 270 | 6 | 39 | 1 | 15 |
| Pepperoni & Cheese | 1 slice | 310 | 8 | 39 | 1 | 19 |
| One Meat w/ Vegetables | 1 slice | 320 | 12 | 38 | 2 | 15 |
| Three Meat w/ Vegetables | 1 slice | 405 | 17 | 40 | 2 | 24 |
| Stuffed Crust Pizza, thick | ... | ... | . | . | . | . |
| Pepperoni & Cheese | 1 slice | 350 | 14 | 39 | 1 | 20 |
| Three Meat w/ Vegetables | 1 slice | 450 | 21 | 40 | 2 | 21 |
| Pizza Rolls, 1 ½", frozen, heated | ... | ... | . | . | . | . |
| With cheese and meat | 5 | 175 | 7 | 20 | 1 | 9 |
| Plantain, without peel | ... | ... | . | . | . | . |
| Fresh, medium size | 1 | 218 | 1 | 57 | 4 | 2 |
| Cooked, slices | 1 cup | 180 | Tr | 48 | 4 | 1 |
| Plum | ... | ... | . | . | . | . |
| Fresh, whole, med, 2 ¼" dia | 1 | 36 | Tr | 9 | 1 | 1 |
| Canned, in heavy syrup | 1 cup | 230 | Tr | 60 | 3 | 1 |
| Canned, in juice | 1 cup | 146 | Tr | 38 | 3 | 1 |
| Pomegranate, avg size, raw | 1 | 105 | 1 | 26 | 2 | 2 |
| Pop Tart – see Toaster Pastry | ... | ... | . | . | . | . |
| Popcorn | ... | ... | . | . | . | . |
| Air popped | 1 cup | 30 | Tr | 6 | 1 | 1 |
| Caramel coated w/ peanuts | 1 cup | 170 | 3 | 34 | 2 | 3 |
| Caramel coated w/o peanuts | 1 cup | 150 | 5 | 28 | 2 | 1 |
| Cheese flavored | 1 cup | 60 | 4 | 6 | 1 | 1 |
| Microwave, butter flavor | 1 cup | 40 | 2 | 4 | 1 | 1 |
| Microwave, butter, reduced fat | 1 cup | 30 | 1 | 5 | 1 | 1 |
| Popped in oil | 1 cup | 55 | 3 | 6 | 1 | 1 |
| Popped in oil, buttered | 1 cup | 75 | 5 | 6 | 1 | 1 |
| Popcorn Cake, plain | 1 | 38 | Tr | 8 | Tr | 1 |
| Butter flavor | 1 | 40 | Tr | 8 | Tr | 1 |
| Carmel | 1 | 48 | Tr | 11 | Tr | 1 |
| Poppyseed pastry filling | 1 Tbsp | 65 | 1 | 14 | 1 | 1 |
| Popsicle – see Frozen Dessert | ... | ... | . | . | . | . |
| **PORK** | ... | ... | . | . | . | . |
| (Weights for meat w/o bones) | ... | ... | . | . | . | . |
| Bacon, regular | 3 slices | 110 | 9 | Tr | 0 | 6 |
| Bacon, Canadian | 3 slices | 125 | 6 | 1 | 0 | 17 |

| FOOD: (See Beverages & Fast Food Restaurants listed separately) | Serv- ing Size | Cal- ories | Fat (g) | Carb (g) | Fi- ber (g) | Pro- tein (g) |
|---|---|---|---|---|---|---|
| Boston Butt, roasted, lean | 3 oz | 205 | 9 | 0 | 0 | 27 |
| Picnic Pork | 3.5 oz | 280 | 21 | Tr | 0 | 20 |
| Pork Chop, loin cut | ... | ... | . | . | . | . |
| broiled, lean & fat | 3 oz | 205 | 11 | 0 | 0 | 24 |
| broiled, lean only | 3 oz | 170 | 7 | 0 | 0 | 26 |
| pan fried, lean & fat | 3 oz | 235 | 14 | 0 | 0 | 25 |
| pan fried, lean only | 3 oz | 195 | 9 | 0 | 0 | 27 |
| Rib Roast, lean & fat | 3 oz | 215 | 13 | 0 | 0 | 23 |
| lean only | 3 oz | 195 | 9 | 0 | 0 | 24 |
| Sausage | ... | ... | . | . | . | . |
| breakfast link, small | 1 link | 70 | 6 | Tr | 0 | 3 |
| breakfast patty, small | 1 patty | 80 | 7 | Tr | 0 | 3 |
| sausage, regular | 2 oz | 120 | 10 | 1 | 0 | 7 |
| sausage, lowfat | 2 oz | 80 | 2 | 6 | 0 | 7 |
| Polish Kielbasa sausage | 2 oz | 120 | 10 | Tr | 0 | 8 |
| Vienna sausage, 2" links | 2 links | 90 | 8 | Tr | 0 | 4 |
| Shoulder cut, braised, lean & fat | 3 oz | 280 | 20 | 0 | 0 | 24 |
| lean only | 3 oz | 210 | 10 | 0 | 0 | 27 |
| Spareribs, braised | 3 oz | 335 | 26 | 0 | 0 | 25 |
| (Other Pork Products, see: | ... | ... | . | . | . | . |
| Bologna, Ham, Hot Dog, | ... | ... | . | . | . | . |
| Salami, & specific entrées) | ... | ... | . | . | . | . |
| Pork Chop, fried | 3 oz | 235 | 14 | 0 | 0 | 25 |
| Marie Callendar entrée | 1 meal | 550 | 27 | 50 | 2 | 26 |
| Pork Rinds, about 1 cup | 1 oz | 155 | 9 | 0 | 0 | 17 |
| Pot Pie, 4" dia, frozen, heated | ... | ... | . | . | . | . |
| Beef Pot Pie | 1 pie | 480 | 27 | 40 | 2 | 19 |
| Chicken Pot Pie | 1 pie | 410 | 23 | 38 | 2 | 11 |
| Turkey Pot Pie | 1 pie | 400 | 22 | 38 | 2 | 11 |
| Pot Roast | ... | ... | . | . | . | . |
| Lean Cuisine entrée | 1 meal | 190 | 6 | 19 | 1 | 15 |
| Marie Callender entrée | 1 meal | 250 | 6 | 31 | 1 | 17 |
| Swanson entrée | 1 meal | 405 | 10 | 48 | 2 | 30 |
| POTATO | ... | ... | . | . | . | . |
| (also see Sweet Potatoes) | ... | ... | . | . | . | . |
| Au Gratin Potatoes | 1 cup | 300 | 16 | 28 | 4 | 9 |
| Baked potato, 4 ¾" x 2 ¼" | ... | ... | . | . | . | . |
| whole potato w/skin | 1 | 220 | Tr | 51 | 5 | 5 |
| whole potato w/o skin | 1 | 145 | Tr | 34 | 2 | 3 |
| Baked, & filled or topped, | ... | ... | . | . | . | . |
| large potato, 6" x 2 ½" | ... | ... | . | . | . | . |

| FOOD: (See Beverages & Fast Food Restaurants listed separately) | Serv-ing Size | Cal-ories | Fat (g) | Carb (g) | Fi-ber (g) | Pro-tein (g) |
|---|---|---|---|---|---|---|
| bacon & cheese | 1 | 530 | 18 | 78 | 5 | 17 |
| broccoli & cheese | 1 | 470 | 14 | 80 | 6 | 9 |
| cheese | 1 | 570 | 23 | 78 | 5 | 14 |
| chili & cheese | 1 | 620 | 24 | 83 | 5 | 20 |
| sour cream & chives | 1 | 390 | 6 | 73 | 6 | 7 |
| Boiled potato, 2 ½" dia | ... | ... | . | . | . | . |
| peeled, whole potato | 1 | 116 | Tr | 27 | 2 | 2 |
| peeled, diced | 1 cup | 134 | Tr | 31 | 3 | 3 |
| French Fries | ... | ... | . | . | . | . |
| Frozen, heated | ... | ... | . | . | . | . |
| thin shoestring strips, 3 oz | 20 fries | 130 | 4 | 22 | 2 | 2 |
| thick or crinkle cut, 4.5 oz | 20 fries | 195 | 6 | 33 | 3 | 3 |
| Restaurant type, medium order | 1 med | 350 | 15 | 48 | 5 | 5 |
| Hash Browns, patty, 3" x 2" | 1 patty | 80 | 9 | 9 | 1 | 2 |
| Hash Browned potatoes | 1 cup | 280 | 14 | 32 | 2 | 4 |
| Mashed, w/milk & margarine | 1 cup | 220 | 9 | 35 | 4 | 4 |
| Scalloped potatoes | 1 cup | 245 | 11 | 29 | 4 | 8 |
| Tater Tots type fried potatoes | 10 pc | 175 | 8 | 24 | 3 | 3 |
| Potato Chips | ... | ... | . | . | . | . |
| (about 14 chips, unless noted) | ... | ... | . | . | . | . |
| Plain, regular | 1 oz | 155 | 10 | 15 | 1 | 2 |
| Barbecue flavor | 1 oz | 155 | 10 | 15 | 1 | 2 |
| Cheddar cheese | 1 oz | 160 | 10 | 15 | 1 | 2 |
| Fat free chips | 1 oz | 75 | Tr | 17 | 1 | 2 |
| Pringles, regular | 1 oz | 160 | 11 | 15 | 1 | 1 |
| Reduced fat chips | 1 oz | 140 | 7 | 18 | 1 | 2 |
| Rippled chips (about 12 chips) | 1 oz | 160 | 10 | 15 | 1 | 2 |
| Ruffles, original (12 chips) | 1 oz | 160 | 10 | 14 | 1 | 2 |
| Ruffles, reduced fat (13 chips) | 1 oz | 140 | 7 | 18 | 1 | 2 |
| Ranch flavor chips | 1 oz | 155 | 10 | 15 | 2 | 2 |
| Sour cream & onion flavor | 1 oz | 155 | 10 | 15 | 2 | 2 |
| Potato Salad | 1 cup | 360 | 21 | 28 | 3 | 7 |
| Potato Sticks, fried, crunchy | 1 cup | 250 | 15 | 26 | 3 | 3 |
| Preserves | ... | ... | . | . | . | . |
| All flavors, regular | 1 Tbsp | 55 | Tr | 14 | Tr | Tr |
| All flavors, restaurant packet | 1 pkt | 39 | Tr | 10 | Tr | Tr |
| Pretzels | ... | ... | . | . | . | . |
| Sticks, regular | 25 | 58 | 1 | 12 | 1 | 1 |
| Mini Twists, regular | 10 | 58 | 1 | 12 | 1 | 1 |
| Bavarian, twisted, 2 ½" x 3" | 1 | 60 | 1 | 13 | 1 | 1 |
| Chocolate coated | 1 oz | 130 | 5 | 20 | 1 | 2 |

| FOOD: (See Beverages & Fast Food Restaurants listed separately) | Serving Size | Calories | Fat (g) | Carb (g) | Fiber (g) | Protein (g) |
|---|---|---|---|---|---|---|
| Dutch, twisted, 2 ½" x 3" | 1 | 60 | 1 | 13 | 1 | 1 |
| Honey Mustard nuggets | 10 | 150 | 4 | 24 | 1 | 3 |
| Soft, twisted, large, 3" x 5" | 1 | 180 | 2 | 36 | 2 | 5 |
| Sourdough, twisted, 2 ½" x 3" | 1 | 60 | 1 | 13 | 1 | 1 |
| Prosciutto, Boars Head | 1 oz | 60 | 3 | 0 | 0 | 8 |
| Prunes, dried, pitted | … | … | . | . | . | . |
| Uncooked, unsweetened | 5 prunes | 100 | Tr | 26 | 3 | 1 |
| Stewed, unsweetened | 1 cup | 265 | 1 | 70 | 16 | 3 |
| Pudding | … | … | … | … | … | … |
| Butterscotch, regular | ½ cup | 150 | 5 | 25 | Tr | 3 |
| Caramel w/chocolate, regular | ½ cup | 150 | 5 | 25 | 1 | 3 |
| Chocolate, regular | ½ cup | 150 | 5 | 25 | 1 | 3 |
| fat free | ½ cup | 105 | Tr | 23 | 1 | 3 |
| sugar free | ½ cup | 110 | 1 | 18 | 1 | 2 |
| Rice pudding, regular | ½ cup | 185 | 8 | 25 | Tr | 2 |
| Tapioca, regular | ½ cup | 135 | 4 | 22 | Tr | 2 |
| fat free | ½ cup | 100 | Tr | 23 | Tr | 2 |
| Vanilla, regular | ½ cup | 145 | 4 | 25 | Tr | 3 |
| fat free | ½ cup | 105 | Tr | 24 | Tr | 2 |
| sugar free | ½ cup | 110 | 1 | 18 | Tr | 2 |
| Pumpkin | … | … | . | . | . | . |
| Fresh, cooked, mashed | 1 cup | 50 | Tr | 12 | 3 | 2 |
| Canned, heated | 1 cup | 83 | 1 | 20 | 7 | 3 |
| Quesadilla | … | … | . | . | . | . |
| Cheese | 1 | 350 | 18 | 31 | 2 | 16 |
| Chicken | 1 | 400 | 19 | 33 | 2 | 25 |
| Radish, fresh, raw, avg 1" dia | 5 | 5 | Tr | 1 | Tr | Tr |
| Raisin | … | … | . | . | . | . |
| Golden or natural, not packed | 1 cup | 435 | 1 | 115 | 6 | 5 |
| Golden or natural, 0.5 oz pkg | 1 pkg | 42 | Tr | 11 | 1 | Tr |
| Golden or natural, not packed | 3 Tbsp | 84 | Tr | 22 | 1 | Tr |
| Raisin Bran – see Cereal | … | … | . | . | . | . |
| Raspberries | … | … | . | . | . | . |
| Fresh | 1 cup | 60 | 1 | 14 | 8 | 1 |
| Frozen, sweetened, thawed | 1 cup | 260 | Tr | 65 | 11 | 2 |
| Ravioli | … | … | . | . | . | . |
| Beef | 1 cup | 255 | 4 | 44 | 1 | 12 |
| Cheese | 1 cup | 265 | 5 | 44 | 1 | 11 |
| Relish – see Pickle Relish or specific listing | … … | … … | . . | . . | . . | . . |
| Rhubarb | … | … | . | . | . | . |

| FOOD:<br>(See Beverages & Fast Food Restaurants listed separately) | Serving Size | Calories | Fat (g) | Carb (g) | Fiber (g) | Protein (g) |
|---|---|---|---|---|---|---|
| Fresh, diced | 1 cup | 28 | Tr | 6 | Tr | Tr |
| Frozen, cooked, sweetened | 1 cup | 278 | Tr | 75 | 5 | 1 |
| **RICE** | ... | ... | . | . | . | . |
| Plain Rice Dishes | ... | ... | . | . | . | . |
| Brown long grain rice, boiled | 1 cup | 215 | 2 | 45 | 4 | 5 |
| Brown long grain, prep w/butter | 1 cup | 315 | 13 | 45 | 4 | 5 |
| Long grain & wild rice, boiled | 1 cup | 200 | 1 | 40 | 3 | 6 |
| Long grain & wild prep w/butter | 1 cup | 300 | 12 | 40 | 3 | 6 |
| White rice, boiled | 1 cup | 200 | Tr | 44 | 1 | 4 |
| White rice, prep w/butter | 1 cup | 300 | 11 | 44 | 1 | 4 |
| Wild rice, boiled | 1 cup | 170 | 1 | 35 | 3 | 7 |
| Wild rice, prep w/butter | 1 cup | 270 | 12 | 35 | 3 | 7 |
| Yellow rice, boiled | 1 cup | 220 | Tr | 49 | 3 | 5 |
| Mixed & Flavored Rice Dishes | ... | ... | . | . | . | . |
| Flavored w/ beef or pork | 1 cup | 280 | 4 | 52 | 3 | 8 |
| Fried rice w/ beef | 1 cup | 295 | 7 | 48 | 3 | 10 |
| Fried rice w/ chicken | 1 cup | 265 | 6 | 44 | 3 | 9 |
| Fried rice w/ pork | 1 cup | 290 | 6 | 48 | 3 | 11 |
| Fried rice w/ shrimp | 1 cup | 260 | 5 | 44 | 3 | 9 |
| Fried rice w/ vegetables | 1 cup | 255 | 4 | 48 | 3 | 7 |
| Rice & beans | 1 cup | 300 | 7 | 49 | 3 | 11 |
| Rice & vegetables | 1 cup | 260 | 3 | 50 | 3 | 8 |
| Rice Pilaf w/vegetables | 1 cup | 240 | 3 | 45 | 3 | 6 |
| Rice-a-Roni | ... | ... | . | . | . | . |
| Beef vermicelli rice dish | 1 cup | 290 | 4 | 51 | 3 | 9 |
| Broccoli & cheddar rice dish | 1 cup | 330 | 8 | 48 | 3 | 10 |
| Cheddar & herbs rice dish | 1 cup | 310 | 7 | 48 | 3 | 10 |
| Chicken & vegetable rice | 1 cup | 290 | 3 | 51 | 3 | 8 |
| Chicken vermicelli rice dish | 1 cup | 290 | 3 | 52 | 3 | 9 |
| Herb & butter rice dish | 1 cup | 280 | 4 | 53 | 3 | 8 |
| Mexican style rice | 1 cup | 265 | 4 | 45 | 3 | 7 |
| Rice pilaf | 1 cup | 305 | 4 | 54 | 3 | 8 |
| Spanish rice dish | 1 cup | 270 | 4 | 45 | 3 | 7 |
| Rice Cake, plain | 1 | 35 | Tr | 7 | Tr | 1 |
| Butter flavor | 1 | 40 | Tr | 8 | Tr | 1 |
| Carmel | 1 | 48 | Tr | 11 | Tr | 1 |
| Rice Krispies Treat | 1 bar | 90 | 2 | 18 | Tr | 1 |
| Rigatoni, meat sauce | ... | ... | . | . | . | . |
| Lean Cuisine entrée | 1 meal | 260 | 10 | 25 | 2 | 18 |
| Roast Beef – see Beef | ... | ... | . | . | . | . |
| Roast Beef Sandwich | ... | ... | . | . | . | . |

| FOOD: (See Beverages & Fast Food Restaurants listed separately) | Serv- ing Size | Cal- ories | Fat (g) | Carb (g) | Fi- ber (g) | Pro- tein (g) |
|---|---|---|---|---|---|---|
| 3 oz meat w/ sauce | 1 avg | 390 | 19 | 33 | 3 | 23 |
| Rolls – see Bread | ... | ... | . | . | . | . |
| Rosemary, dried spice | ½ tsp | 2 | 0 | Tr | Tr | Tr |
| Rutabaga, cubed, cooked | 1 cup | 65 | Tr | 15 | 3 | 2 |
| Saccharin sweetener | 1 pkt | 0 | 0 | Tr | 0 | 0 |
| Sage, dried spice | ½ tsp | 1 | 0 | Tr | Tr | Tr |
| **SALAD DRESSING** | ... | ... | . | . | . | . |
| Blue cheese, regular | 1 Tbsp | 75 | 8 | 1 | 0 | 1 |
| Blue cheese, low calorie | 1 Tbsp | 15 | 1 | 1 | 0 | 1 |
| Buttermilk, regular | 1 Tbsp | 60 | 6 | 1 | 0 | Tr |
| Buttermilk, low calorie | 1 Tbsp | 15 | 1 | 1 | 0 | Tr |
| Caesar, regular | 1 Tbsp | 80 | 8 | Tr | Tr | Tr |
| Caesar, low calorie | 1 Tbsp | 17 | 1 | 3 | Tr | Tr |
| French, regular | 1 Tbsp | 70 | 6 | 3 | 0 | Tr |
| French, low calorie | 1 Tbsp | 25 | 1 | 4 | 0 | Tr |
| Honey Dijon, regular | 1 Tbsp | 70 | 6 | 3 | 0 | Tr |
| Honey Dijon, fat free | 1 Tbsp | 25 | 1 | 4 | 0 | Tr |
| Italian, regular | 1 Tbsp | 70 | 7 | 1 | 0 | Tr |
| Italian, low calorie | 1 Tbsp | 16 | 1 | 1 | 0 | Tr |
| Mayonnaise, regular | 1 Tbsp | 100 | 11 | Tr | 0 | Tr |
| Mayonnaise, light | 1 Tbsp | 50 | 5 | 1 | 0 | Tr |
| Mayonnaise, fat free | 1 Tbsp | 10 | 0 | 2 | 0 | Tr |
| Ranch, regular | 1 Tbsp | 70 | 6 | 2 | 0 | Tr |
| Ranch, low calorie | 1 Tbsp | 20 | 1 | 3 | 0 | Tr |
| Russian, regular | 1 Tbsp | 75 | 8 | 2 | 0 | Tr |
| Russian, low calorie | 1 Tbsp | 25 | 1 | 4 | Tr | Tr |
| Thousand island, regular | 1 Tbsp | 65 | 6 | 2 | 0 | Tr |
| Thousand island, low calorie | 1 Tbsp | 26 | 2 | 2 | Tr | Tr |
| Zero Carb Salad Dressing | ... | ... | . | . | . | . |
| Nature's Flavors | ... | ... | . | . | . | . |
| Carbfree Blue Cheese | 2 Tbsp | 30 | 3 | 0 | 0 | 1 |
| Carbfree French | 2 Tbsp | 30 | 3 | 0 | 0 | 1 |
| Salad, Tossed | ... | ... | . | . | . | . |
| All Vegetable salad, no dressing | 1 ½ cup | 60 | Tr | 11 | 4 | 3 |
| Salad w/egg & cheese | ... | ... | . | . | . | . |
| no dressing | 1 ½ cup | 120 | 7 | 5 | 1 | 9 |
| w/regular dressing, any type | 1 ½ cup | 200 | 17 | 6 | 1 | 10 |
| w/light dressing, any type | 1 ½ cup | 135 | 7 | 9 | 1 | 9 |
| Salad w/grilled chicken or turkey | ... | ... | . | . | . | . |
| no dressing | 1 ½ cup | 150 | 3 | 11 | 1 | 19 |
| w/regular dressing, any type | 1 ½ cup | 250 | 13 | 12 | 1 | 20 |

| FOOD: (See Beverages & Fast Food Restaurants listed separately) | Serv-ing Size | Cal-ories | Fat (g) | Carb (g) | Fi-ber (g) | Pro-tein (g) |
|---|---|---|---|---|---|---|
| w/light dressing, any type | 1 ½ cup | 175 | 3 | 15 | 1 | 19 |
| (Also see Pasta Salad, Potato | ... | ... | . | . | . | . |
| Salad, & specific listings) | ... | ... | . | . | . | . |
| Salami | ... | ... | . | . | . | . |
| Regular, any meat | 2 oz | 130 | 11 | 1 | 0 | 7 |
| Lowfat, Turkey or Chicken, | ... | ... | . | . | . | . |
| thin 1/8" slices | 2 slices | 80 | 5 | 1 | 0 | 8 |
| Cotto | 2 slices | 95 | 7 | 1 | 0 | 7 |
| Dried type, 3" x 1/8" slices | 2 slices | 95 | 7 | 1 | 0 | 6 |
| Hard | 1 oz | 110 | 9 | 1 | 0 | 6 |
| Salisbury Steak | ... | ... | . | ... | . | . |
| Banquet entrée | 1 meal | 220 | 16 | 8 | 1 | 9 |
| Morton's entrée | 1 meal | 210 | 9 | 23 | 2 | 9 |
| Stouffer's entrée | 1 meal | 240 | 15 | 10 | 1 | 17 |
| Weight Watchers entrée | 1 meal | 150 | 9 | 24 | 1 | 19 |
| Salsa | 1 Tbsp | 4 | Tr | 1 | Tr | Tr |
| Salt | ... | ... | . | . | . | . |
| Regular | ½ tsp | 0 | 0 | 0 | 0 | 0 |
| Reduced sodium | ½ tsp | 0 | 0 | 0 | 0 | 0 |
| Seasoned | ½ tsp | 5 | Tr | Tr | Tr | Tr |
| Sandwich, (w/ 3 oz Meat on | ... | ... | . | . | . | . |
| Lg 6" bun, sub, or kaiser roll) | ... | ... | . | . | . | . |
| Cold Cuts, mixed meats w/ | ... | ... | . | .. | . | . |
| sauce, cheese, tomato, lettuce | 1 | 455 | 19 | 51 | 2 | 22 |
| Ham & Cheese w/ sauce | 1 | 495 | 23 | 53 | 2 | 23 |
| Roast Beef w/ mayo, tomato, | ... | ... | . | . | . | . |
| lettuce | 1 | 498 | 23 | 53 | 2 | 24 |
| Tuna salad w/ mayo, lettuce | 1 | 585 | 28 | 55 | 2 | 30 |
| Sandwich Meat, see Lunch Meat | ... | ... | . | . | . | . |
| Sandwich Spread | 1 Tbsp | 35 | 3 | 2 | Tr | 1 |
| SAUCE | ... | ... | . | . | . | . |
| A1 Steak Sauce | 1 Tbsp | 15 | 0 | 3 | Tr | 0 |
| Barbecue sauce, regular | 1 Tbsp | 20 | Tr | 4 | 1 | Tr |
| Barbecue, thick or honey | 1 Tbsp | 40 | 1 | 8 | Tr | Tr |
| Catsup | 1 Tbsp | 18 | Tr | 4 | Tr | Tr |
| Cheese sauce | ¼ cup | 110 | 8 | 4 | Tr | 4 |
| Chili sauce | ¼ cup | 60 | Tr | 13 | 3 | 1 |
| Duck Sauce | 1 Tbsp | 20 | 0 | 4 | Tr | 0 |
| Hoison sauce | 1 Tbsp | 35 | 1 | 7 | Tr | 1 |
| Hollandaise sauce | 1 Tbsp | 18 | 1 | 2 | Tr | 1 |
| Horseradish, prepared | 1 tsp | 4 | Tr | 1 | Tr | Tr |

| FOOD: (See Beverages & Fast Food Restaurants listed separately) | Serv-ing Size | Cal-ories | Fat (g) | Carb (g) | Fi-ber (g) | Pro-tein (g) |
|---|---|---|---|---|---|---|
| Hot sauce | 1 tsp | 1 | Tr | Tr | Tr | Tr |
| Marinara sauce | ¼ cup | 36 | 1 | 5 | 1 | 1 |
| Mayonnaise, regular | 1 Tbsp | 100 | 11 | Tr | 0 | Tr |
| Mayonnaise, light | 1 Tbsp | 50 | 5 | 1 | 0 | Tr |
| Mayonnaise, fat free | 1 Tbsp | 10 | 0 | 2 | 0 | Tr |
| Mustard, regular | 1 tsp | 4 | Tr | Tr | Tr | Tr |
| Mustard, hot or honey | 1 tsp | 8 | Tr | 2 | Tr | Tr |
| Oyster sauce | 1 Tbsp | 5 | Tr | 1 | Tr | Tr |
| Pasta sauce | ¼ cup | 35 | 1 | 5 | 1 | 1 |
| Pepper sauce, hot | 1 tsp | 1 | Tr | Tr | Tr | Tr |
| Pickle Relish | 1 Tbsp | 20 | Tr | 5 | Tr | Tr |
| Pizza sauce | ¼ cup | 35 | 1 | 5 | 1 | 1 |
| Salsa | 1 Tbsp | 4 | Tr | 1 | Tr | Tr |
| Sloppy Joe sauce w/meat | 1 Tbsp | 45 | 2 | 5 | 1 | 2 |
| Soy sauce | 1 Tbsp | 10 | Tr | 1 | Tr | 1 |
| Spaghetti sauce | ¼ cup | 36 | 1 | 5 | 1 | 1 |
| Steak Sauce | 1 Tbsp | 15 | 0 | 3 | Tr | 0 |
| Sweet & Sour Sauce | 1 Tbsp | 20 | 0 | 4 | Tr | 0 |
| Szechuan sauce | 1 Tbsp | 20 | Tr | 3 | Tr | 1 |
| Tabasco sauce | 1 tsp | 1 | Tr | Tr | Tr | Tr |
| Taco sauce | 1 Tbsp | 10 | Tr | 2 | Tr | Tr |
| Tamari Sauce | 1 Tbsp | 11 | 0 | 1 | 0 | 2 |
| Tartar sauce | 1 Tbsp | 45 | 4 | 2 | Tr | 0 |
| Teriyaki sauce | 1 Tbsp | 20 | Tr | 4 | Tr | 1 |
| Tomato sauce | ½ cup | 37 | Tr | 9 | 2 | 1 |
| White sauce | ¼ cup | 92 | 6 | 6 | Tr | 3 |
| Worcestershire sauce | 1 Tbsp | 12 | 0 | 3 | Tr | 0 |
| Zero Carb Sauce | … | … | . | . | . | . |
| Nature's Flavors | … | … | . | . | . | . |
| Barbecue sauce | 2 Tbsp | 0 | 0 | 0 | 0 | 0 |
| Honey Mustard sauce | 2 Tbsp | 0 | 0 | 0 | 0 | 0 |
| Sauerkraut | 1 cup | 45 | Tr | 10 | 6 | 2 |
| **Sausage** | … | … | . | . | . | . |
| Breakfast link, small | 1 link | 70 | 6 | Tr | 0 | 3 |
| Breakfast patty, small | 1 patty | 80 | 7 | Tr | 0 | 3 |
| Beef or Pork sausage | 2 oz | 120 | 10 | 1 | 0 | 7 |
| Chicken or Turkey sausage | 2 oz | 98 | 8 | 1 | 0 | 6 |
| Lowfat sausage, beef or pork | 2 oz | 80 | 2 | 6 | 0 | 7 |
| Lowfat sausage, chicken or turkey | 2 oz | 78 | 2 | 6 | 0 | 7 |
| Fat free sausage, beef or pork | 2 oz | 60 | 0 | 6 | 0 | 7 |
| Fat free sausage, | … | … | . | . | . | . |

| FOOD:<br>(See Beverages & Fast Food Restaurants listed separately) | Serving Size | Calories | Fat (g) | Carb (g) | Fiber (g) | Protein (g) |
|---|---|---|---|---|---|---|
| chicken or turkey | 2 oz | 58 | 0 | 6 | 0 | 7 |
| Polish sausage, Kielbasa | 2 oz | 120 | 10 | Tr | 0 | 8 |
| Vienna sausage, 2" links | 2 links | 90 | 8 | Tr | 0 | 4 |
| Scallop - see Fish/Seafood | … | … | . | . | . | . |
| Seafood – see Fish/Seafood | … | … | . | . | . | . |
| Seasoning – see specific listings | … | … | . | . | . | . |
| Blended Seasoning w/ salt, | … | … | . | . | . | . |
| garlic, onion, paprika, papain | ½ tsp | 2 | 0 | Tr | Tr | Tr |
| Seaweed | … | … | . | . | . | . |
| Kelp, raw | 2 Tbsp | 4 | Tr | 1 | Tr | Tr |
| Spirulina, dried | 1 Tbsp | 3 | Tr | Tr | Tr | 1 |
| Thin wrap sheets | 1 sheet | 10 | Tr | 2 | Tr | 1 |
| Seeds | … | … | . | . | . | . |
| Pumpkin seeds, roasted | 1 oz | 148 | 12 | 4 | 1 | 9 |
| Sesame seeds, plain | 1 Tbsp | 47 | 4 | 1 | Tr | 2 |
| Sesame seeds, butter, roasted | 1 Tbsp | 90 | 8 | 3 | 1 | 3 |
| Soybean seeds, dried, boiled | ½ cup | 145 | 7 | 9 | 5 | 15 |
| Sunflower seeds, dry roasted | 1 oz | 165 | 14 | 7 | 3 | 5 |
| (Also see specific listings) | … | … | . | . | . | . |
| Shallot, raw, chopped | 1 Tbsp | 7 | Tr | 2 | Tr | Tr |
| Shark – see Fish | … | … | . | . | . | . |
| Sherbet, Orange | ½ cup | 100 | 1 | 22 | 0 | 1 |
| Sherbet, Rainbow | ½ cup | 105 | 1 | 23 | 0 | 1 |
| Shortening, regular cottonseed & | 1 cup | 1810 | 205 | 0 | 0 | 0 |
| soybean blend | 1 Tbsp | 115 | 13 | 0 | 0 | 0 |
| Shrimp – see Fish/Seafood | … | … | . | . | . | . |
| & specific entrées | … | … | . | . | . | . |
| Shrimp & Broccoli | … | … | . | . | . | . |
| w/creamy white sauce | 1 cup | 270 | 10 | 29 | 1 | 15 |
| Shrimp & Pasta | … | … | . | . | . | . |
| w/creamy white sauce | 1 cup | 300 | 13 | 34 | 1 | 14 |
| Shrimp & Vegetables | … | … | . | . | . | . |
| Hunan style | 1 cup | 240 | 7 | 30 | 3 | 14 |
| Shrimp & Vegetables | … | … | . | . | . | . |
| w/szechuan sauce | 1 cup | 230 | 6 | 30 | 3 | 14 |
| Shrimp Marinara | … | … | . | . | . | . |
| Weight Watchers entrée | 1 meal | 200 | 2 | 37 | 1 | 8 |
| Sirloin Steak – see Beef | … | … | . | . | . | . |
| Snack Mix, Chex Mix | ¾ cup | 120 | 5 | 18 | 2 | 3 |
| Sorbet, orange or raspberry | ½ cup | 120 | 0 | 30 | 0 | 0 |

| FOOD: (See Beverages & Fast Food Restaurants listed separately) | Serv- ing Size | Cal- ories | Fat (g) | Carb (g) | Fi- ber (g) | Pro- tein (g) |
|---|---|---|---|---|---|---|
| Soufflé, regular type | 1 cup | 250 | 20 | 3 | 1 | 12 |
| **SOUP**   (as prep) | … | … | . | . | . | . |
| Bouillon cube, regular, | … | … | . | . | . | . |
| all varieties, makes 1 cup | 1 cube | 5 | Tr | 1 | Tr | Tr |
| Bouillon packet, low sodium, | … | … | . | . | . | . |
| all varieties, makes 1 cup | 1 pkt | 15 | Tr | 3 | Tr | Tr |
| Broth, consommé, all varieties | 1 cup | 20 | Tr | 3 | Tr | 1 |
| Bean w/ Ham soup | 1 cup | 185 | 7 | 24 | 9 | 8 |
| Bean w/ Pork soup | 1 cup | 175 | 6 | 23 | 9 | 8 |
| Beef Noodle soup | 1 cup | 83 | 3 | 9 | 1 | 5 |
| Chicken Noodle soup, regular | 1 cup | 75 | 2 | 9 | 1 | 4 |
| Chicken Noodle soup, chunky | 1 cup | 175 | 6 | 17 | 4 | 13 |
| Chicken & Rice soup | 1 cup | 70 | 2 | 8 | 1 | 5 |
| Chicken & Vegetable, regular | 1 cup | 90 | 1 | 12 | 1 | 6 |
| Chicken & Vegetable, chunky | 1 cup | 165 | 5 | 19 | 1 | 12 |
| Clam Chowder, Manhattan | 1 cup | 85 | 2 | 12 | 2 | 2 |
| Clam Chowder, New England | 1 cup | 165 | 7 | 17 | 2 | 9 |
| Clam Chowder, Low fat, | … | … | . | . | . | . |
| New England | 1 cup | 115 | 2 | 20 | 1 | 5 |
| Cream of Broccoli soup | … | … | . | . | . | . |
| prep w/ water | 1 cup | 125 | 9 | 8 | 1 | 2 |
| prep w/ milk | 1 cup | 195 | 14 | 14 | 1 | 6 |
| Cream of Chicken soup | … | … | . | . | . | . |
| prep w/ water | 1 cup | 117 | 7 | 9 | Tr | 3 |
| prep w/ milk | 1 cup | 190 | 11 | 15 | Tr | 7 |
| Cream of Mushroom soup | … | … | . | . | . | . |
| prep w/ water | 1 cup | 130 | 9 | 9 | 1 | 2 |
| prep w/ milk | 1 cup | 200 | 14 | 15 | 1 | 6 |
| Lentil soup, low fat | 1 cup | 125 | 2 | 20 | 6 | 8 |
| Minestrone | 1 cup | 85 | 3 | 11 | 1 | 4 |
| Onion soup | 1 cup | 100 | 2 | 19 | 4 | 4 |
| Pea soup | 1 cup | 160 | 3 | 26 | 3 | 9 |
| Potato w/ bean soup | 1 cup | 170 | 7 | 23 | 2 | 6 |
| Ramen Beef Noodle soup | 1 cup | 190 | 8 | 26 | 1 | 4 |
| Ramen Chicken noodle soup | 1 cup | 190 | 8 | 26 | 1 | 4 |
| Ramen Mushroom noodle soup | 1 cup | 180 | 7 | 26 | 1 | 4 |
| Tomato soup, prep w/ water | 1 cup | 85 | 2 | 17 | 1 | 2 |
| Tomato soup, prep w/ milk | 1 cup | 160 | 6 | 22 | 1 | 6 |
| Vegetable soup | 1 cup | 72 | 2 | 12 | 1 | 2 |
| Vegetable Beef soup | 1 cup | 90 | 2 | 11 | 1 | 7 |
| Wisconsin Cheese soup | 1 cup | 280 | 18 | 20 | 2 | 10 |

| FOOD:<br>(See Beverages & Fast Food Restaurants listed separately) | Serving Size | Calories | Fat (g) | Carb (g) | Fiber (g) | Protein (g) |
|---|---|---|---|---|---|---|
| Sour cream | … | … | . | . | . | . |
| Regular | 1 cup | 495 | 48 | 10 | 0 | 7 |
| Regular | 1 Tbsp | 25 | 3 | 1 | 0 | Tr |
| Reduced fat | 1 Tbsp | 20 | 2 | 1 | 0 | Tr |
| Fat free | 1 Tbsp | 12 | 0 | 2 | 0 | Tr |
| Soy Burger, broiled | 1 patty | 100 | 1 | 9 | 3 | 15 |
| Soybeans | … | … | . | . | . | . |
| dried mature seeds, cooked | ½ cup | 145 | 7 | 9 | 5 | 15 |
| Spaghetti | … | … | . | . | . | . |
| Plain, cooked | 1 cup | 195 | 1 | 40 | 2 | 7 |
| With cheese & tomato sauce | 1 cup | 220 | 2 | 41 | 3 | 8 |
| With meatballs in tomato sauce | 1 cup | 240 | 4 | 41 | 3 | 7 |
| With tomato sauce | 1 cup | 260 | 10 | 31 | 3 | 11 |
| Spaghetti Bolognese, w/ meat sauce, Healthy Choice entrée | …<br>1 meal | …<br>255 | .<br>3 | .<br>43 | .<br>5 | .<br>14 |
| Spare Ribs – see Pork | … | … | . | . | . | . |
| Spice – see specific listings | … | … | . | . | . | . |
| Blended Spice w/ basil, garlic, oregano, rosemary, thyme | …<br>½ tsp | …<br>3 | .<br>0 | .<br>Tr | .<br>Tr | .<br>Tr |
| Spinach | … | … | . | . | . | . |
| Fresh, raw, chopped | 1 cup | 7 | Tr | 1 | Tr | 1 |
| Fresh, chopped, cooked | 1 cup | 41 | Tr | 7 | 4 | 5 |
| Frozen, chopped, cooked | 1 cup | 53 | Tr | 10 | 6 | 6 |
| Canned, cooked | 1 cup | 50 | Tr | 7 | 5 | 6 |
| Spinach Soufflé | 1 cup | 220 | 18 | 3 | 1 | 11 |
| Spread | … | … | . | . | . | . |
| Cheese Spread | 1 Tbsp | 40 | 3 | 1 | 0 | 3 |
| Sandwich Spread | 1 Tbsp | 35 | 3 | 2 | Tr | 1 |
| (also see spreads in Margarine) | … | … | . | . | . | . |
| Squash | … | … | . | . | . | . |
| Butternut squash | ¾ cup | 150 | 6 | 25 | 4 | 2 |
| Summer, raw, sliced | 1 cup | 23 | Tr | 5 | 2 | 1 |
| Summer, cooked, slices | 1 cup | 36 | 1 | 8 | 3 | 2 |
| Winter, baked, cubes | 1 cup | 80 | 1 | 18 | 6 | 2 |
| Winter, frozen, cooked, mashed | 1 cup | 94 | Tr | 24 | 2 | 3 |
| Squash Casserole | ¾ cup | 330 | 24 | 20 | 6 | 7 |
| Steak – see Beef | … | … | . | . | . | . |
| Steak Sauce, A1 | 1 Tbsp | 15 | 0 | 3 | Tr | 0 |
| Strawberries | … | … | . | . | . | . |
| Fresh, medium size, 1 ¼" dia | 10 | 40 | Tr | 9 | 3 | 1 |

| FOOD:  (See Beverages & Fast Food Restaurants listed separately) | Serv-ing Size | Cal-ories | Fat (g) | Carb (g) | Fi-ber (g) | Pro-tein (g) |
|---|---|---|---|---|---|---|
| Fresh, sliced | 1 cup | 50 | 1 | 12 | 4 | 1 |
| Frozen, sweetened, thawed | 1 cup | 245 | Tr | 66 | 5 | 1 |
| Strawberry Shortcake | 1 avg | 275 | 15 | 20 | 2 | 6 |
| Streusel  (avg size slice) | … | … | . | . | . | . |
| Apple | 1 slice | 240 | 17 | 33 | 2 | 4 |
| Cherry | 1 slice | 205 | 16 | 30 | 2 | 4 |
| Stuffing, as prep | … | … | . | . | . | . |
| Traditional stuffing, seasoned,  meat flavored | … 1 cup | … 360 | . 18 | . 44 | . 6 | . 6 |
| Corn bread stuffing, seasoned | 1 cup | 345 | 17 | 42 | 5 | 5 |
| Succotash | ½ cup | 80 | 1 | 17 | 3 | 3 |
| **Sugar** | … | … | . | . | . | . |
| White, regular, granulated | … | … | . | . | . | . |
| One cup | 1 cup | 774 | 0 | 200 | 0 | 0 |
| One tablespoon | 1 Tbsp | 45 | 0 | 12 | 0 | 0 |
| One teaspoon | 1 tsp | 15 | 0 | 4 | 0 | 0 |
| Restaurant size packet | 1 pkt | 24 | 0 | 6 | 0 | 0 |
| White, Confectioner's, Powdered | … | … | . | . | . | . |
| Unsifted, one cup | 1 cup | 31 | 0 | 8 | 0 | 0 |
| Unsifted, one tablespoon | 1 Tbsp | 467 | 0 | 119 | 0 | 0 |
| Brown Sugar | … | … | . | . | . | . |
| Packed, one cup | 1 cup | 827 | 0 | 214 | 0 | 0 |
| Not packed , one cup | 1 cup | 545 | 0 | 141 | 0 | 0 |
| Not packed, one tablespoon | 1 Tbsp | 34 | 0 | 9 | 0 | 0 |
| Sugar Substitute | … | … | . | . | . | . |
| Aspartame – Equal, Nutrasweet | 1 pkt | 0 | 0 | Tr | 0 | 0 |
| Saccharine - Sweet & Low | 1 pkt | 0 | 0 | Tr | 0 | 0 |
| Sucralose - Splenda | 1 pkt | 0 | 0 | Tr | 0 | 0 |
| Sundae  (small serving) | … | … | . | . | . | . |
| Hot Fudge | 1 | 285 | 9 | 48 | 1 | 6 |
| Strawberry | 1 | 230 | 3 | 45 | 1 | 6 |
| Strawberry Yogurt | 1 | 275 | 1 | 59 | 1 | 9 |
| Swedish Meatballs | … | … | . | . | . | . |
| Celentano, 6 meatball meal | 1 meal | 260 | 19 | 5 | Tr | 12 |
| Lean Cuisine entrée | 1 meal | 290 | 7 | 35 | 1 | 22 |
| Weight Watchers entrée | 1 meal | 290 | 7 | 34 | 1 | 18 |
| Sweet 'N Low | 1 pkt | 0 | 0 | Tr | 0 | 0 |
| Sweet Potato | … | … | . | . | . | . |
| Baked w/skin 4" x 2" | 1 whole | 165 | Tr | 38 | 4 | 3 |
| Baked or Boiled w/o skin 4" x 2" | 1 whole | 150 | Tr | 35 | 3 | 3 |

| FOOD:  (See Beverages & Fast Food Restaurants listed separately) | Serv- ing Size | Cal- ories | Fat (g) | Carb (g) | Fi- ber (g) | Pro- tein (g) |
|---|---|---|---|---|---|---|
| Boiled, peeled, mashed | ½ cup | 170 | 3 | 30 | 3 | 3 |
| Candied, 2 ½" x 2" pieces | 1 piece | 145 | 3 | 29 | 3 | 1 |
| Canned in syrup, drained | 1 cup | 210 | 1 | 50 | 6 | 3 |
| Canned, vacuum pack, mashed | 1 cup | 230 | 1 | 54 | 5 | 4 |
| Whipped, frozen, heated | ½ cup | 140 | 6 | 18 | 3 | 2 |
| Sweet Potato Casserole | ¾ cup | 280 | 18 | 39 | 4 | 3 |
| Sweet Roll - see specific listings | ... | ... | . | . | . | . |
| Syrup | ... | ... | . | . | . | . |
| Butterscotch | 1 Tbsp | 60 | 1 | 12 | Tr | 0 |
| Chocolate, thin | 1 Tbsp | 55 | Tr | 12 | Tr | Tr |
| Chocolate fudge, thick | 1 Tbsp | 65 | 2 | 12 | 1 | 1 |
| Corn, light | 1 Tbsp | 56 | 0 | 15 | 0 | 0 |
| Maple | 1 Tbsp | 52 | Tr | 13 | 0 | 0 |
| Molasses, blackstrap | 1 Tbsp | 47 | 0 | 12 | 0 | 0 |
| Pancake Syrup/Table Syrup | ... | ... | . | . | . | . |
| Regular | 1 Tbsp | 55 | 0 | 14 | 0 | 0 |
| Light, reduced calorie | 1 Tbsp | 25 | 0 | 7 | 0 | 0 |
| Sugar free | 1 Tbsp | 8 | 0 | 3 | Tr | 0 |
| Zero Carb Syrup | ... | ... | . | . | . | . |
| Nature's Flavors | ... | ... | . | . | . | . |
| Apple | 2 Tbsp | 0 | 0 | 0 | 0 | 0 |
| Brown Sugar | 2 Tbsp | 0 | 0 | 0 | 0 | 0 |
| Chocolate | 2 Tbsp | 0 | 0 | 0 | 0 | 0 |
| Maple | 1 Tbsp | 0 | 0 | 0 | 0 | 0 |
| Taco  (w/hard or soft shell) | ... | ... | . | . | . | . |
| Regular size, with beef | 1 | 210 | 11 | 18 | 2 | 11 |
| Regular size, with chicken | 1 | 190 | 8 | 17 | 2 | 13 |
| Large, with steak or beef | 1 | 280 | 17 | 20 | 2 | 13 |
| X-Lg, double decker, with beef | 1 | 365 | 18 | 27 | 2 | 21 |
| Taco Salad w/ ground beef, cheese, taco shell | ... 1 | ... 275 | . 15 | . 24 | . 2 | . 13 |
| Taco Shell   (shell only) | ... | ... | . | . | . | . |
| Thin shell, 6" dia | 1 | 60 | 3 | 8 | 1 | 1 |
| Large shell | 1 | 100 | 5 | 13 | 1 | 2 |
| Tahini, from toasted kernels | 1 Tbsp | 90 | 8 | 3 | 1 | 3 |
| Tamale,  meatless | 2 pc | 215 | 8 | 30 | 1 | 6 |
| Beef, Swanson entrée | 1 meal | 350 | 13 | 46 | 1 | 13 |
| Chicken, Swanson entrée | 1 meal | 325 | 12 | 45 | 1 | 8 |
| Tangerine, fresh, med, 2 ½" dia | 1 | 37 | Tr | 9 | 2 | 1 |
| Tapioca, pearl, dry | 1 cup | 545 | Tr | 135 | 1 | Tr |
| Taro Leaf, steamed | ½ cup | 18 | Tr | 4 | 2 | 1 |

| FOOD: (See Beverages & Fast Food Restaurants listed separately) | Serv- ing Size | Cal- ories | Fat (g) | Carb (g) | Fi- ber (g) | Pro- tein (g) |
|---|---|---|---|---|---|---|
| Tarragon, ground | 1 tsp | 5 | Tr | 1 | Tr | Tr |
| Tater Tots  fried potatoes | 10 | 175 | 8 | 24 | 3 | 3 |
| T-bone Steak – see Beef | … | … | . | . | . | . |
| Teriyaki – see Beef Teriyaki or   Chicken Teriyaki | … … | … … | . . | . . | . . | . . |
| Thyme, dried spice | ½ tsp | 2 | 0 | Tr | Tr | Tr |
| Toaster Pastry  (Pop Tart) | … | … | . | . | . | . |
| Apple, frosted | 1 pastry | 200 | 5 | 37 | 1 | 2 |
| Apple, unfrosted | 1 pastry | 185 | 5 | 34 | 1 | 2 |
| Blueberry, frosted | 1 pastry | 200 | 5 | 37 | 1 | 2 |
| Blueberry, unfrosted | 1 pastry | 185 | 5 | 34 | 1 | 2 |
| Brown sugar, cinnamon, frosted | 1 pastry | 190 | 5 | 36 | 1 | 2 |
| Chocolate, frosted | 1 pastry | 200 | 5 | 37 | 1 | 3 |
| Chocolate fudge, frosted | 1 pastry | 200 | 5 | 36 | 1 | 3 |
| Grape, frosted | 1 pastry | 200 | 5 | 37 | 1 | 2 |
| Grape, unfrosted | 1 pastry | 185 | 5 | 34 | 1 | 2 |
| Lowfat, frosted, any variety | 1 pastry | 170 | 2 | 37 | 1 | 2 |
| Lowfat, unfrosted, any variety | 1 pastry | 155 | 2 | 33 | 1 | 2 |
| S'mores, frosted | 1 pastry | 220 | 6 | 39 | 1 | 2 |
| Strawberry, frosted | 1 pastry | 200 | 5 | 37 | 1 | 2 |
| Strawberry, unfrosted | 1 pastry | 185 | 5 | 34 | 1 | 2 |
| Tofu, plain, cooked, 4 oz | ½ cup | 80 | 4 | 2 | Tr | 9 |
| Tomatillos, raw, medium size | 2 | 22 | Tr | 4 | 1 | Tr |
| Tomato | … | … | . | . | . | . |
| Fresh, raw, avg size 2 ½" dia | 1 whole | 26 | Tr | 6 | 1 | 1 |
| Fresh, raw, cherry tomato | 1 whole | 4 | Tr | 1 | Tr | Tr |
| Fresh, slices, ¼" thick | 1 slice | 4 | Tr | 1 | Tr | Tr |
| Fresh, chopped or sliced | 1 cup | 38 | 1 | 8 | 2 | 2 |
| Canned, liquids and solids | 1 cup | 46 | Tr | 10 | 2 | 2 |
| Stewed, fresh or canned | 1 cup | 70 | 1 | 17 | 3 | 2 |
| Sun Dried | … | … | . | . | . | . |
| Plain | 1 piece | 5 | Tr | 1 | Tr | Tr |
| Packed in oil, drained | 1 piece | 6 | Tr | 1 | Tr | Tr |
| Tomato Paste | 1 cup | 215 | 1 | 51 | 11 | 10 |
| Tomato Puree | 1 cup | 100 | Tr | 24 | 5 | 4 |
| Tomato Sauce | 1 cup | 74 | Tr | 18 | 3 | 3 |
| Topping,  for dessert | … | … | . | . | . | . |
| Butterscotch, regular | 1 Tbsp | 60 | 1 | 12 | Tr | 0 |
| Butterscotch, light | 1 Tbsp | 30 | Tr | 8 | Tr | 0 |
| Chocolate, regular | 1 Tbsp | 50 | Tr | 11 | 1 | 1 |

| FOOD: (See Beverages & Fast Food Restaurants listed separately) | Serving Size | Calories | Fat (g) | Carb (g) | Fiber (g) | Protein (g) |
|---|---|---|---|---|---|---|
| Chocolate, light | 1 Tbsp | 25 | Tr | 7 | Tr | Tr |
| Cream, Whipped Topping | ... | ... | . | . | . | . |
| Light cream | 1 cup | 700 | 75 | 7 | 0 | 5 |
| Light cream | 1 Tbsp | 45 | 5 | Tr | 0 | Tr |
| Heavy cream | 1 cup | 820 | 88 | 7 | 0 | 5 |
| Heavy cream | 1 Tbsp | 50 | 6 | Tr | 0 | Tr |
| Pressurized in can | 1 Tbsp | 8 | 1 | Tr | 0 | Tr |
| Marshmallow Topping | 1 Tbsp | 50 | Tr | 12 | Tr | Tr |
| Strawberry Topping | 1 Tbsp | 50 | Tr | 11 | Tr | 1 |
| Tortellini | ... | ... | . | . | . | . |
| Cheese filling | 1 cup | 270 | 7 | 40 | 2 | 12 |
| Meat filling | 1 cup | 340 | 9 | 55 | 1 | 21 |
| Spinach filling | 1 cup | 235 | 5 | 30 | 2 | 12 |
| Tortellini Salad w/dressing | ¾ cup | 350 | 24 | 24 | 5 | 11 |
| Tortilla, 6" dia, ready to cook | ... | ... | . | . | . | . |
| Corn | 1 | 60 | 1 | 12 | 1 | 1 |
| Flour | 1 | 105 | 2 | 18 | 1 | 3 |
| Tortilla Chips | ... | ... | . | . | . | . |
| Regular | 1 oz | 140 | 7 | 18 | 2 | 2 |
| Lowfat, baked | 1 oz | 115 | 1 | 22 | 2 | 4 |
| Nacho flavor, regular | 1 oz | 140 | 7 | 18 | 2 | 2 |
| Nacho flavor, reduced fat, baked | 1 oz | 125 | 4 | 20 | 1 | 2 |
| (also see Corn Chips) | ... | ... | . | . | . | . |
| Tostada | ... | ... | . | . | . | . |
| Beef, bean, & cheese | 1 | 330 | 17 | 30 | 2 | 16 |
| Chicken & cheese | 1 | 250 | 11 | 26 | 1 | 15 |
| Guacamole | 1 | 180 | 12 | 16 | 1 | 6 |
| Trail Mix | ... | ... | . | . | . | . |
| Regular w/raisins, nuts, seeds, | ... | ... | . | . | . | . |
| & chocolate chips | 1 cup | 705 | 47 | 66 | 9 | 21 |
| Tropical dried fruit mix | 1 cup | 570 | 24 | 92 | 11 | 9 |
| Tuna – see Fish | ... | ... | . | . | . | . |
| Tuna Dishes | ... | ... | . | . | . | . |
| Tuna & broccoli w/creamy sauce | 1 cup | 300 | 12 | 31 | 1 | 14 |
| Tuna & noodle casserole | 1 cup | 320 | 10 | 37 | 2 | 20 |
| Tuna & pasta w/cheese sauce | 1 cup | 300 | 11 | 36 | 1 | 14 |
| Tuna & pasta w/creamy sauce | 1 cup | 300 | 12 | 36 | 1 | 14 |
| Tuna au gratin | 1 cup | 310 | 12 | 36 | 1 | 14 |
| Tuna fettuccine alfredo | 1 cup | 310 | 14 | 32 | 1 | 14 |
| Tuna romanoff | 1 cup | 280 | 8 | 38 | 1 | 15 |
| Tuna tetrazzini | 1 cup | 310 | 12 | 33 | 1 | 17 |

| FOOD:  (See Beverages & Fast Food Restaurants listed separately) | Serv- ing Size | Cal- ories | Fat (g) | Carb (g) | Fi- ber (g) | Pro- tein (g) |
|---|---|---|---|---|---|---|
| Tuna Salad | ... | ... | . | . | . | . |
| Prep w/tuna in oil, regular | ... | ... | . | . | . | . |
| mayo dressing, pickle relish | ½ cup | 190 | 10 | 9 | 0 | 16 |
| Prep w/ tuna in water, light | ... | ... | . | . | . | . |
| mayo dressing, pickle relish | ½ cup | 130 | 5 | 6 | 0 | 15 |
| **TURKEY** | ... | ... | . | . | . | . |
| Fried Turkey patty, battered | 3 oz | 250 | 15 | 14 | Tr | 12 |
| Roast Turkey | ... | ... | . | . | . | . |
| light & dark meat | 3 oz | 145 | 5 | 3 | 0 | 22 |
| light meat only | 3 oz | 135 | 4 | 0 | 0 | 25 |
| dark meat only | 3 oz | 160 | 6 | 0 | 0 | 25 |
| Giblets, simmered, chopped | 1 cup | 240 | 7 | 3 | 0 | 39 |
| Ground Turkey | 4 oz | 195 | 11 | 0 | 0 | 22 |
| Neck, simmered | 4 oz | 155 | 6 | 0 | 0 | 23 |
| (Other Turkey Products, see: | ... | ... | . | . | . | . |
| Bologna, Hot Dog, Salami, | ... | ... | . | . | . | . |
| Sausage & specific entrées) | ... | ... | . | . | . | . |
| Turkey & Gravy | ... | ... | . | . | . | . |
| Banquet entrée | 1 meal | 140 | 9 | 6 | Tr | 8 |
| Turkey Dijon | ... | ... | . | . | . | . |
| Lean Cuisine entrée | 1 meal | 280 | 10 | 21 | 1 | 26 |
| Turkey Tetrazzini | ... | ... | . | . | . | . |
| Stouffers entrée | 1 meal | 360 | 17 | 33 | 1 | 19 |
| Turmeric, ground | ½ tsp | 4 | Tr | 1 | Tr | Tr |
| Turnip, sliced, cooked | ½ cup | 20 | Tr | 4 | Tr | 1 |
| Turnip Greens, cooked | ½ cup | 16 | Tr | 3 | Tr | 1 |
| Turnover | ... | ... | . | . | . | . |
| Apple or Cherry, large | 1 | 410 | 16 | 63 | 4 | 4 |
| Apple, small | 1 | 170 | 8 | 21 | 2 | 2 |
| Blueberry, small | 1 | 165 | 8 | 23 | 2 | 2 |
| Cherry, small | 1 | 175 | 8 | 21 | 2 | 2 |
| Vanilla Extract | 1 tsp | 12 | Tr | 1 | 0 | Tr |
| Veal | ... | ... | . | . | . | . |
| Chop, loin, braised | 3.5 oz | 285 | 17 | 0 | 0 | 30 |
| Cutlet, braised, lean & fat | 3 oz | 180 | 5 | 0 | 0 | 31 |
| Liver, braised | 3.5 oz | 165 | 7 | 0 | 0 | 22 |
| Rib, roasted, lean & fat | 3.5 oz | 250 | 13 | 0 | 0 | 24 |
| Veal Marsala, Le Menu entrée | 1 meal | 250 | 5 | 25 | 1 | 25 |
| Veal Parmagiana | ... | ... | . | . | . | . |
| Le Menu entrée | 1 meal | 175 | 6 | 9 | Tr | 22 |

| FOOD: (See Beverages & Fast Food Restaurants listed separately) | Serving Size | Calories | Fat (g) | Carb (g) | Fiber (g) | Protein (g) |
|---|---|---|---|---|---|---|
| Morton entrée | 1 meal | 280 | 13 | 30 | 1 | 8 |
| Vegetable Burger, broiled | 1 patty | 100 | 1 | 9 | 4 | 15 |
| Vegetables, mixed | ... | ... | . | . | . | . |
| (See specific listings for | ... | ... | . | . | . | . |
| individual vegetables) | ... | ... | . | . | . | . |
| Mixed, canned, drained, heated | 1 cup | 80 | Tr | 15 | 5 | 4 |
| Mixed, frozen, w/o sauce, heated | ... | ... | . | . | . | . |
| Small vegetables- peas, carrots, | ... | ... | . | . | . | . |
| beans, corn | 1 cup | 105 | Tr | 21 | 5 | 5 |
| Large vegetable cuts- broccoli, | ... | ... | . | . | . | . |
| cauliflower, mushrooms | 1 cup | 27 | 0 | 4 | 3 | 3 |
| Large vegetable cuts | ... | ... | . | . | . | . |
| prep w/ butter sauce | 1 cup | 107 | 9 | 4 | 3 | 3 |
| Vegetables, mixed, Birdseye | ... | ... | . | . | . | . |
| French style | ¾ cup | 110 | 2 | 10 | 3 | 6 |
| Italian style | ½ cup | 100 | 6 | 11 | 3 | 2 |
| Japanese style | ½ cup | 90 | 5 | 10 | 3 | 2 |
| Mexican style | ½ cup | 140 | 5 | 24 | 3 | 5 |
| Oriental style | ½ cup | 60 | 4 | 4 | 2 | 2 |
| Vinegar | ... | ... | . | . | . | . |
| Regular | 1 Tbsp | 2 | 0 | 1 | 0 | 0 |
| Cider vinegar | 1 Tbsp | 2 | 0 | 1 | 0 | 0 |
| Waffle | ... | ... | . | . | . | . |
| Regular, prep from recipe, 7" dia | 1 piece | 215 | 11 | 25 | 1 | 6 |
| Frozen, toaster size, 4 " dia | 1 piece | 90 | 3 | 13 | 1 | 2 |
| Lowfat, toaster size, 4" dia | 1 piece | 80 | 1 | 15 | Tr | 2 |
| Walnut – see Nuts | ... | ... | . | . | . | . |
| Water Chestnut, canned, slices | 1 cup | 75 | Tr | 17 | 4 | 1 |
| Watercress, raw | ½ cup | 2 | 0 | Tr | Tr | Tr |
| Watermelon | ... | ... | . | . | . | . |
| Fresh, diced | 1 cup | 50 | 1 | 11 | 1 | 1 |
| Fresh, wedge, 1" thick, 1/16 of | ... | ... | . | . | . | . |
| melon 15" long x 7 ½" dia | 1 wedge | 92 | 1 | 21 | 1 | 2 |
| Wheat Bran | ¼ cup | 25 | 1 | 3 | 1 | 2 |
| Wheat Germ, toasted, plain | 1 Tbsp | 27 | 1 | 3 | 1 | 2 |
| Whipped Cream – see Cream | ... | ... | . | . | . | . |
| Wiener – see Hot Dog | ... | ... | . | . | . | . |
| Yam – see Sweet Potato | ... | ... | . | . | . | . |
| Yeast | ... | ... | . | . | . | . |
| Compressed | 1 cake | 18 | Tr | 3 | 1 | 1 |

| FOOD: (See Beverages & Fast Food Restaurants listed separately) | Serv-ing Size | Cal-ories | Fat (g) | Carb (g) | Fi-ber (g) | Pro-tein (g) |
|---|---|---|---|---|---|---|
| Dry, active, regular size pkg | 1 pkg | 21 | Tr | 3 | 2 | 3 |
| Dry, active | 1 tsp | 12 | Tr | 2 | 1 | 2 |
| Yogurt | ... | ... | . | . | . | . |
|   Chocolate, regular | ½ cup | 120 | 4 | 18 | 2 | 3 |
|   Chocolate, fat free | ½ cup | 90 | 0 | 17 | 1 | 5 |
|   Strawberry, regular | ½ cup | 120 | 4 | 19 | Tr | 4 |
|   Strawberry, fat free | ½ cup | 100 | 0 | 23 | 0 | 3 |
|   Vanilla, regular | ½ cup | 120 | 4 | 18 | 0 | 3 |
|   Vanilla, fat free | ½ cup | 110 | 0 | 23 | 0 | 4 |
|   Yogurt, plain, | ... | ... | . | . | . | . |
|     made w/ whole milk | ½ cup | 140 | 7 | 11 | 0 | 8 |
|     made w/ lowfat milk | ½ cup | 130 | 3 | 19 | 0 | 11 |
|     made w/ skim milk | ½ cup | 120 | 0 | 15 | 0 | 13 |
|   Yogurt w/fruit, regular varieties | ½ cup | 135 | 3 | 20 | 1 | 5 |
|   Yogurt, w/fruit flavor, sugarfree | ½ cup | 95 | Tr | 16 | 0 | 9 |
| Ziti w/ Meat Sauce | ... | ... | . | . | . | . |
|   Swanson entrée | 1 meal | 560 | 23 | 58 | 1 | 28 |
| Zucchini | ... | ... | . | . | . | . |
|   Fresh, avg size | 1 | 5 | 0 | 1 | Tr | Tr |
|   Sliced, cooked | ½ cup | 15 | 0 | 4 | 1 | Tr |
|   Breaded, fried | ½ cup | 165 | 9 | 16 | 2 | 4 |

# FAST FOOD RESTAURANTS

| FAST FOOD RESTAURANT: (See other Foods and Beverages listed separately) | Serv-ing Size | Cal-ories | Fat (g) | Carb (g) | Fi-ber (g) | Pro-tein (g) |
|---|---|---|---|---|---|---|
| **Arby's** | ... | ... | . | . | . | . |
|   Apple turnover | 1 | 330 | 14 | 48 | 0 | 4 |
|   Arby-Q | 1 | 430 | 18 | 48 | 3 | 22 |
|   Arby's melt w/ cheddar | 1 | 370 | 18 | 36 | 2 | 18 |
|   Arby's sauce | 1 svg | 15 | Tr | 4 | 0 | Tr |
|   Bacon cheddar deluxe | 1 | 540 | 34 | 38 | 3 | 22 |
|   Baked potato, deluxe | 1 | 735 | 36 | 86 | 7 | 19 |

| FAST FOOD RESTAURANT: (See other Foods and Beverages listed separately) | Serving Size | Calories | Fat (g) | Carb (g) | Fiber (g) | Protein (g) |
|---|---|---|---|---|---|---|
| Baked potato, plain | 1 | 355 | Tr | 82 | 7 | 7 |
| Baked potato w/sour cream | 1 | 580 | 24 | 85 | 7 | 9 |
| Barbecue sauce | 1 svg | 30 | 0 | 7 | 0 | 0 |
| Beef & cheddar sandwich | 1 | 490 | 28 | 40 | 2 | 25 |
| Beefstock Au Jus | 1 | 10 | 0 | 1 | 0 | 0 |
| Biscuit, plain | 1 | 280 | 15 | 34 | 1 | 6 |
| Bleu cheese dressing | 1 svg | 290 | 31 | 2 | 0 | 2 |
| Blueberry muffin | 1 | 230 | 9 | 35 | 0 | 2 |
| Boston clam chowder | 1 svg | 190 | 9 | 18 | 1 | 9 |
| Breaded chicken fillet | 1 | 542 | 28 | 46 | 5 | 28 |
| Broccoli & cheddar baked potato | 1 | 580 | 20 | 89 | 9 | 14 |
| Butterfinger polar swirl | 1 | 455 | 18 | 62 | 0 | 15 |
| Cheddar cheese sauce | 1 svg | 35 | 3 | 1 | 0 | 1 |
| Cheddar curly fries | 1 svg | 335 | 18 | 40 | 3 | 3 |
| Cheesecake, plain | 1 | 320 | 23 | 23 | 1 | 5 |
| Cherry turnover | 1 | 320 | 13 | 46 | 1 | 4 |
| Chicken Cordon Bleu | 1 | 625 | 33 | 46 | 5 | 38 |
| Chicken fingers, 2 pieces/svg | 1 svg | 290 | 16 | 20 | 1 | 16 |
| Chocolate chip cookie | 1 | 125 | 6 | 16 | Tr | 2 |
| Chocolate shake | med | 450 | 12 | 76 | 0 | 15 |
| Cinnamon nut Danish | 1 | 360 | 11 | 60 | 1 | 6 |
| Cream of broccoli soup | 1 svg | 160 | 8 | 15 | 2 | 7 |
| Croissant, plain | 1 | 220 | 12 | 25 | 0 | 4 |
| Curly fries | 1 svg | 300 | 15 | 38 | 0 | 4 |
| Fish fillet | 1 | 530 | 27 | 50 | 2 | 23 |
| French dip | 1 svg | 475 | 22 | 40 | 3 | 30 |
| French fries | 1 | 240 | 13 | 30 | 3 | 2 |
| French toast stix, 6 pieces/svg | 1 svg | 430 | 21 | 52 | 3 | 10 |
| Garden salad w/o dressing | 1 | 60 | Tr | 12 | 5 | 3 |
| Grilled chicken deluxe | 1 | 430 | 20 | 41 | 3 | 23 |
| Grilled chicken barbecue | 1 | 390 | 13 | 47 | 2 | 23 |
| Ham & cheese | 1 | 355 | 14 | 24 | 2 | 24 |
| Ham & cheese melt | 1 | 335 | 13 | 34 | 2 | 20 |
| Heath polar swirl | 1 | 545 | 22 | 76 | 0 | 15 |
| Honey French dressing | 1 svg | 275 | 23 | 18 | 0 | 0 |
| Horsey sauce | 1 svg | 55 | 5 | 2 | 0 | 0 |
| Hot ham & Swiss | 1 | 500 | 23 | 43 | 2 | 30 |
| Italian sub sandwich | 1 | 670 | 36 | 46 | 2 | 30 |
| Italian sub sauce | 1 svg | 70 | 7 | 1 | 0 | 0 |
| Jamocha shake | small | 385 | 10 | 62 | 0 | 15 |
| Junior roast beef | 1 | 325 | 14 | 35 | 2 | 17 |

| FAST FOOD RESTAURANT: (See other Foods and Beverages listed separately) | Serv-ing Size | Cal-ories | Fat (g) | Carb (g) | Fi-ber (g) | Pro-tein (g) |
|---|---|---|---|---|---|---|
| Light mayonnaise | 1 svg | 12 | 1 | 1 | Tr | 0 |
| Lumberjack mixed vegetables | 1 svg | 90 | 4 | 10 | 1 | 2 |
| Old fashion chicken noodle soup | 1 svg | 80 | 2 | 11 | 1 | 6 |
| Oreo polar swirl | 1 | 480 | 22 | 66 | 1 | 15 |
| Parmesan cheese sauce | 1 svg | 70 | 7 | 1 | 0 | 0 |
| Peanut butter cup polar swirl | 1 | 515 | 24 | 61 | 1 | 20 |
| Philly beef & Swiss | 1 | 750 | 47 | 48 | 3 | 39 |
| Potato cakes | 1 svg | 200 | 12 | 20 | 2 | 2 |
| Potato with bacon soup | 1 svg | 170 | 7 | 23 | 2 | 6 |
| Red ranch dressing | 1 svg | 75 | 6 | 5 | 0 | 0 |
| Reduced cal honey mayonnaise | 1 svg | 70 | 7 | 1 | 0 | 0 |
| Reduced calorie Italian dressing | 1 svg | 20 | 1 | 3 | 0 | 0 |
| Reduced cal buttermilk ranch | 1 svg | 50 | Tr | 12 | 0 | 0 |
| Roast beef sandwich, regular | 1 | 390 | 19 | 33 | 3 | 23 |
| Roast beef deluxe sandwich | 1 | 300 | 10 | 33 | 6 | 18 |
| Roast beef sub sandwich | 1 | 700 | 42 | 44 | 4 | 38 |
| Roast chicken club | 1 | 545 | 31 | 37 | 2 | 31 |
| Roast chicken Santa Fe | 1 | 435 | 22 | 35 | 1 | 29 |
| Roast chicken deluxe | 1 | 280 | 6 | 33 | 4 | 20 |
| Roast chicken salad | 1 | 150 | 2 | 12 | 5 | 20 |
| Roast turkey deluxe | 1 | 260 | 7 | 33 | 4 | 20 |
| Side salad w/o dressing | 1 | 25 | Tr | 4 | 2 | 1 |
| Snickers polar swirl | 1 | 510 | 19 | 73 | 1 | 15 |
| Super roast beef | 1 | 525 | 27 | 50 | 5 | 15 |
| Timberline chili | 1 svg | 220 | 10 | 17 | 7 | 18 |
| Triple cheese melt | 1 | 720 | 45 | 46 | 2 | 37 |
| Turkey sub sandwich | 1 | 550 | 27 | 47 | 2 | 31 |
| Vanilla shake | small | 360 | 12 | 50 | 0 | 15 |
| Wisconsin cheese soup | 1 svg | 280 | 18 | 20 | 2 | 10 |
| **Baskin Robbins** | ... | ... | . | . | . | . |
| Aloha berry banana smoothie | 1 | 165 | Tr | 36 | 1 | 3 |
| Bora berry smoothie | 1 | 175 | Tr | 38 | 2 | 4 |
| Café mocha yogurt | 1 | 80 | Tr | 15 | 1 | 4 |
| Calypso berry smoothie | 1 | 160 | Tr | 35 | 2 | 3 |
| Chocolate chip ice cream | 1 | 155 | 9 | 16 | Tr | 2 |
| Chocolate chocolate chip, sugarfree | ... | ... | . | . | . | . |
| | 1 | 100 | 3 | 17 | Tr | 4 |
| Chocolate ice cream | 1 | 155 | 8 | 19 | Tr | 3 |
| Chocolate yogurt | 1 | 80 | 0 | 15 | 1 | 5 |
| Copa banana smoothie | 1 | 145 | Tr | 30 | 1 | 4 |
| Daiquiri ice | 1 | 110 | 0 | 27 | 0 | 0 |

| FAST FOOD RESTAURANT: (See other Foods and Beverages listed separately) | Serv-ing Size | Cal-ories | Fat (g) | Carb (g) | Fi-ber (g) | Pro-tein (g) |
|---|---|---|---|---|---|---|
| Dutch chocolate | 1 | 105 | Tr | 23 | 1 | 4 |
| Espresso & cream | 1 | 110 | 4 | 18 | 0 | 3 |
| Maui brownie madness | 1 | 145 | 3 | 26 | 1 | 5 |
| Perils of praline | 1 | 130 | 3 | 24 | 0 | 4 |
| Rainbow sherbet | 1 | 120 | 2 | 25 | 0 | 1 |
| Raspberry cheese Louise | 1 | 135 | 3 | 24 | 0 | 4 |
| Red raspberry sorbet | 1 | 120 | 0 | 30 | 0 | 0 |
| Rocky road ice cream | 1 | 165 | 8 | 21 | Tr | 3 |
| Silk chocolate | 1 | 120 | 0 | 25 | 1 | 5 |
| Strawberry yogurt, nonfat | 1 | 105 | 0 | 23 | 0 | 3 |
| Sunset orange smoothie | 1 | 150 | Tr | 32 | 2 | 4 |
| Thin mint, sugarfree | 1 | 100 | 3 | 17 | 0 | 4 |
| Tropic of fruit yogurt, nonfat | 1 | 130 | 0 | 28 | 0 | 4 |
| Tropical tango smoothie | 1 | 180 | Tr | 40 | 1 | 4 |
| Vanilla bean dream yogurt, nonfat | ... 1 | ... 110 | . 0 | . 23 | . 0 | . 4 |
| Vanilla bean dream | 1 | 120 | 0 | 25 | 0 | 5 |
| Vanilla chocolate twist, nonfat | 1 | 100 | 0 | 21 | 1 | 4 |
| Vanilla ice cream | 1 | 145 | 8 | 14 | 0 | 3 |
| Vanilla yogurt | 1 | 80 | 0 | 15 | 1 | 4 |
| Very berry strawberry ice cream | 1 | 120 | 6 | 16 | 0 | 2 |
| **Boston Market** | ... | ... | . | . | . | . |
| Apples w/ cinnamon | 1 svg | 252 | 5 | 56 | 3 | Tr |
| Barbecue baked beans | 1 svg | 330 | 9 | 53 | 9 | 11 |
| Black beans with rice | 1 svg | 300 | 10 | 45 | 5 | 8 |
| Broccoli and rice casserole | 1svg | 240 | 12 | 26 | 3 | 5 |
| Brownie, chocolate | 1 | 310 | 10 | 51 | 3 | 3 |
| Cake, chocolate | 1 piece | 505 | 24 | 73 | 2 | 3 |
| Cake, hummingbird | 1 piece | 705 | 36 | 92 | 2 | 6 |
| Carrots, glazed | 1 svg | 280 | 15 | 35 | 2 | 1 |
| Cheesecake | 1 piece | 575 | 41 | 44 | 1 | 9 |
| Chicken with skin, ½ | 1 | 625 | 37 | 2 | 0 | 70 |
| Chicken w/o skin, ¼, dark meat | 1 | 210 | 10 | 1 | 0 | 28 |
| Chicken with skin, ¼, dark meat | 1 | 325 | 22 | 2 | 0 | 30 |
| Chicken w/o skin, ¼, white meat | 1 | 165 | 4 | 1 | 0 | 31 |
| Chicken w/ skin, ¼, white meat | 1 | 310 | 17 | 2 | 0 | 43 |
| Chicken Caesar salad | 1 | 670 | 47 | 16 | 2 | 45 |
| Chicken pot pie | 1 | 745 | 46 | 57 | 3 | 26 |
| Chicken salad sandwich | 1 | 675 | 30 | 63 | 3 | 39 |
| Chicken sandwich | 1 | 390 | 5 | 60 | 2 | 31 |
| Chicken sandwich, barbecued | 1 | 540 | 9 | 84 | 2 | 30 |

| FAST FOOD RESTAURANT: (See other Foods and Beverages listed separately) | Serv- ing Size | Cal- ories | Fat (g) | Carb (g) | Fi- ber (g) | Pro- tein (g) |
|---|---|---|---|---|---|---|
| Chicken sandwich w/cheese | 1 | 630 | 28 | 61 | 2 | 37 |
| Cole slaw | 1 svg | 300 | 19 | 30 | 3 | 2 |
| Cookie, chocolate chip | 1 | 390 | 19 | 33 | 2 | 3 |
| Cookie, oatmeal | 1 | 390 | 20 | 47 | 2 | 5 |
| Cookie, peanut butter | 1 | 420 | 25 | 43 | 2 | 7 |
| Corn, buttered w/herbs | 1 svg | 180 | 4 | 30 | 2 | 5 |
| Corn, whole kernel | 1 svg | 180 | 4 | 30 | 2 | 5 |
| Cornbread | 1 svg | 200 | 6 | 33 | 2 | 3 |
| Cranberry relish | 1 svg | 330 | 5 | 70 | 2 | 1 |
| Cranberry walnut relish | 1 svg | 365 | 6 | 75 | 3 | 3 |
| Green beans | 1 svg | 80 | 6 | 5 | 3 | 1 |
| Green bean casserole | 1 svg | 85 | 5 | 9 | 3 | 1 |
| Ham with honey glaze | 5 oz | 210 | 8 | 10 | 1 | 24 |
| Ham sandwich | 1 | 410 | 8 | 65 | 2 | 25 |
| Ham sandwich w/cheese & sauce | 1 | 655 | 31 | 67 | 2 | 31 |
| Macaroni and cheese | 1 svg | 280 | 11 | 33 | 3 | 13 |
| Meatloaf | 5 oz | 290 | 17 | 15 | 1 | 20 |
| Meatloaf sandwich w/ cheese | 1 | 695 | 27 | 83 | 3 | 36 |
| Meatloaf sandwich, open faced | 1 | 730 | 36 | 74 | 2 | 29 |
| Pie, apple streusel | 1 piece | 480 | 18 | 63 | 2 | 4 |
| Pie, cherry streusel | 1 piece | 410 | 17 | 60 | 2 | 4 |
| Pie, pecan | 1 piece | 555 | 27 | 71 | 3 | 5 |
| Pie, pumpkin | 1 piece | 370 | 17 | 50 | 2 | 5 |
| Potatoes, dill & garlic | 1 svg | 130 | 3 | 25 | 2 | 3 |
| Potatoes, mashed | 1 svg | 185 | 8 | 25 | 2 | 3 |
| Potatoes, mashed w/gravy | 1 svg | 205 | 9 | 27 | 2 | 4 |
| Potatoes, new | 1 svg | 130 | 3 | 25 | 2 | 3 |
| Potato salad | 1 svg | 200 | 12 | 22 | 2 | 3 |
| Red beans and rice | 1 svg | 260 | 5 | 45 | 3 | 8 |
| Rice pilaf | 1 svg | 180 | 5 | 32 | 2 | 5 |
| Salad, Caesar | 1 svg | 200 | 17 | 7 | 2 | 7 |
| Salad, chunky chicken | 1 svg | 480 | 39 | 4 | 1 | 25 |
| Salad, cucumber | 1 svg | 120 | 10 | 9 | 3 | 2 |
| Salad, fruit | 1 svg | 70 | 1 | 15 | 3 | 1 |
| Salad, tortellini | 1 svg | 350 | 24 | 24 | 3 | 11 |
| Spinach, creamed | 1 svg | 260 | 20 | 11 | 3 | 9 |
| Squash, butternut | 1 svg | 160 | 6 | 25 | 3 | 2 |
| Squash casserole | 1 svg | 335 | 24 | 20 | 2 | 7 |
| Stuffing, savory | 1 svg | 310 | 12 | 44 | 2 | 6 |
| Sweet potato casserole | 1 svg | 280 | 18 | 39 | 3 | 3 |
| Turkey bacon club sandwich | 1 | 780 | 38 | 64 | 3 | 47 |

| FAST FOOD RESTAURANT: (See other Foods and Beverages listed separately) | Serving Size | Calories | Fat (g) | Carb (g) | Fiber (g) | Protein (g) |
|---|---|---|---|---|---|---|
| Turkey breast w/o skin | 5 oz | 170 | 1 | 1 | 0 | 36 |
| Turkey sandwich, regular | 1 | 390 | 4 | 61 | 2 | 33 |
| Turkey sandwich w/cheese | 1 | 615 | 25 | 64 | 2 | 39 |
| Turkey sandwich, open faced | 1 | 715 | 20 | 64 | 2 | 47 |
| Vegetables, steamed, w/o sauce | 1 svg | 35 | 1 | 7 | 3 | 2 |
| Zucchini marinara | 1 svg | 80 | 4 | 10 | 2 | 2 |
| **Burger King** | ... | ... | . | . | . | . |
| A.M. express dip | 1 svg | 85 | Tr | 21 | 2 | 2 |
| A.M. express grape jam | 1 svg | 30 | 0 | 7 | Tr | 0 |
| A.M. express strawberry jam | 1 svg | 30 | 0 | 8 | Tr | 0 |
| Bacon bits | 1 svg | 15 | 1 | 0 | 0 | 1 |
| Barbecue sauce | 1 svg | 35 | Tr | 9 | 0 | 0 |
| Barbecue sauce, bull's eye | 1 svg | 20 | Tr | 5 | 0 | 0 |
| Biscuit with sausage | 1 | 585 | 40 | 41 | 1 | 16 |
| Biscuit w/ bacon, egg & cheese | 1 | 510 | 31 | 39 | 1 | 19 |
| BK big fish | 1 | 695 | 41 | 56 | 3 | 26 |
| BK broiler | 1 | 550 | 29 | 41 | 2 | 30 |
| Bleu cheese dressing | 1 svg | 160 | 16 | 1 | 0 | 2 |
| Broiled chicken salad | 1 | 200 | 10 | 7 | 3 | 21 |
| Cheeseburger | 1 | 385 | 19 | 28 | 1 | 23 |
| Chicken sandwich | 1 | 705 | 43 | 54 | 2 | 26 |
| Chicken tenders, 8 pieces/svg | 1 svg | 310 | 17 | 19 | 3 | 3 |
| Chocolate shake | med | 445 | 7 | 84 | 2 | 2 |
| Croissanwich with sausage, egg & cheese | ... ... 1 | ... 600 | . 46 | . 25 | . 1 | . 1 |
| Croutons | 1 svg | 30 | 1 | 4 | 0 | Tr |
| Double cheeseburger | 1 | 605 | 36 | 28 | 1 | 1 |
| Double cheeseburger w/ bacon | 1 | 640 | 39 | 28 | 1 | 1 |
| Double whopper | 1 | 875 | 56 | 45 | 3 | 3 |
| Double whopper w/ cheese | 1 | 965 | 63 | 46 | 3 | 3 |
| Dutch apple pie | 1 | 300 | 15 | 39 | 2 | 2 |
| French dressing | 1 svg | 145 | 10 | 11 | 0 | Tr |
| French fries | med | 375 | 20 | 43 | 3 | 3 |
| French fries, coated | med | 340 | 17 | 43 | 3 | 3 |
| French toast sticks | 1 svg | 505 | 27 | 60 | 1 | 1 |
| Garden salad w/o dressing | 1 | 100 | 5 | 7 | 3 | 3 |
| Hamburger | 1 | 335 | 15 | 28 | 1 | 1 |
| Hash browns | 1 | 220 | 12 | 25 | 2 | 2 |
| Honey dressing | 1 svg | 90 | Tr | 23 | Tr | Tr |
| Land o'lakes classic whip blend | 1 svg | 65 | 7 | 0 | 0 | 0 |
| Onion rings | 1 svg | 315 | 14 | 41 | 6 | 6 |

| FAST FOOD RESTAURANT: (See other Foods and Beverages listed separately) | Serv- ing Size | Cal- ories | Fat (g) | Carb (g) | Fi- ber (g) | Pro- tein (g) |
|---|---|---|---|---|---|---|
| Ranch dressing | 1 svg | 175 | 17 | 2 | 0 | 0 |
| Reduced calorie Italian dressing | 1 svg | 15 | 1 | 3 | 0 | 0 |
| Side salad w/o dressing | 1 | 60 | 3 | 4 | 2 | 2 |
| Strawberry shake | med | 425 | 6 | 93 | 1 | 1 |
| Sweet & sour sauce | 1 svg | 45 | 0 | 11 | 0 | 0 |
| Tartar sauce | 1 svg | 145 | 12 | 7 | 0 | 0 |
| Thousand island dressing | 1 svg | 180 | 19 | 0 | 0 | 0 |
| Vanilla shake | med | 305 | 6 | 54 | 3 | 3 |
| Whopper junior | 1 | 425 | 24 | 29 | 2 | 2 |
| Whopper junior w/ cheese | 1 | 460 | 28 | 29 | 2 | 2 |
| Whopper | 1 | 645 | 38 | 45 | 3 | 3 |
| Whopper w/ cheese | 1 | 735 | 45 | 46 | 3 | 3 |
| Chinese Restaurant – see Panda Express Chinese Food | ... ... | ... ... | . . | . . | . . | . . |
| **Dairy Queen** (all listings regular size, unless noted) | ... ... ... | ... ... ... | . . . | . . . | . . . | . . . |
| Banana split | 1 | 515 | 12 | 96 | 3 | 8 |
| Buster bar | 1 | 445 | 28 | 41 | 2 | 10 |
| Butterfinger blizzard | 1 | 750 | 26 | 115 | 1 | 16 |
| Caramel & nut bar | 1 | 260 | 13 | 32 | 1 | 5 |
| Chocolate cone | 1 | 360 | 11 | 56 | 1 | 9 |
| Chocolate soft serve | ½ cup | 150 | 5 | 22 | 1 | 4 |
| Chocolate dilly bar | 1 | 450 | 28 | 21 | 1 | 3 |
| Chocolate dilly bar, mint | 1 | 190 | 12 | 20 | 1 | 3 |
| Chocolate malt | 1 | 880 | 22 | 155 | 1 | 18 |
| Chocolate shake | 1 | 770 | 20 | 130 | 2 | 17 |
| Chocolate sundae | 1 | 410 | 10 | 73 | 1 | 8 |
| Cookie dough blizzard | 1 | 945 | 36 | 142 | 2 | 17 |
| Dipped cone | 1 | 515 | 25 | 63 | 1 | 9 |
| DQ frozen heart cake | 1 piece | 270 | 9 | 41 | 2 | 5 |
| DQ frozen log cake | 1 piece | 280 | 9 | 43 | 2 | 5 |
| DQ frozen round cake | 1 piece | 340 | 12 | 53 | 2 | 7 |
| DQ frozen sheet cake | 1 piece | 350 | 12 | 54 | 2 | 7 |
| DQ fudge bar | 1 | 60 | Tr | 13 | Tr | 3 |
| DQ lemon freez'r | 1 | 80 | 0 | 20 | Tr | 0 |
| DQ orange bar | 1 | 60 | 0 | 15 | Tr | Tr |
| DQ sandwich | 1 | 150 | 5 | 24 | 1 | 3 |
| DQ vanilla orange bar | 1 | 60 | 0 | 17 | Tr | 2 |
| DQ vanilla soft serve | ½ cup | 140 | 5 | 22 | Tr | 3 |
| DQ yogurt, nonfat frozen | ½ cup | 100 | 0 | 21 | Tr | 3 |

| FAST FOOD RESTAURANT: (See other Foods and Beverages listed separately) | Serving Size | Calories | Fat (g) | Carb (g) | Fiber (g) | Protein (g) |
|---|---|---|---|---|---|---|
| Fudge nut bar | 1 | 410 | 25 | 40 | 2 | 8 |
| Heath blizzard | 1 | 818 | 33 | 119 | 2 | 14 |
| Heath breeze | 1 | 710 | 18 | 123 | 2 | 15 |
| Heath treatzza pizza | 1 slice | 180 | 7 | 28 | 2 | 3 |
| M&M treatzza pizza | 1 slice | 190 | 7 | 29 | 2 | 3 |
| Misty slush | 1 | 290 | 0 | 74 | Tr | 0 |
| Oreo blizzard | 1 | 640 | 23 | 79 | 2 | 10 |
| Peanut buster parfait | 1 | 730 | 31 | 99 | 2 | 16 |
| Peanut butter fudge treatzza pizza | 1 slice | 220 | 10 | 28 | 2 | 4 |
| Queen's choice choc. big scoop | 1 | 250 | 14 | 28 | 2 | 4 |
| Queen's choice vanilla big scoop | 1 | 250 | 14 | 27 | Tr | 4 |
| Reeses peanut butter cup blizzard | 1 | 785 | 33 | 105 | 2 | 19 |
| Starkiss | 1 | 80 | 0 | 21 | Tr | 0 |
| Strawberry blizzard | 1 | 570 | 16 | 95 | 1 | 12 |
| Strawberry breeze | 1 | 460 | 1 | 99 | 1 | 13 |
| Strawberry misty cooler | 1 piece | 190 | 0 | 49 | Tr | 0 |
| Strawberry shortcake | 1 | 430 | 14 | 24 | 2 | 7 |
| Toffee dilly bar | 1 | 210 | 12 | 24 | 1 | 3 |
| Vanilla cone | 1 | 355 | 10 | 57 | 0 | 8 |
| Vanilla cone, small | 1 | 230 | 7 | 38 | 0 | 6 |
| Yogurt cone | 1 | 280 | 1 | 59 | 1 | 9 |
| Yogurt cup | 1 | 230 | 1 | 49 | 1 | 8 |
| Yogurt strawberry sundae | 1 | 305 | 1 | 66 | 1 | 10 |
| **Denny's** | ... | ... | . | . | . | . |
| Banana split | 1 | 885 | 43 | 121 | 3 | 15 |
| Biscuit with sausage gravy | 7 oz | 395 | 21 | 45 | 2 | 8 |
| Buffalo wings, 12 per svg | 1 svg | 855 | 54 | 1 | Tr | 92 |
| Carrots with honey glaze | 1 svg | 80 | 3 | 12 | 2 | 1 |
| Charleston chicken dinner | 1 | 325 | 18 | 16 | 1 | 25 |
| Cheesecake | 1 slice | 470 | 27 | 48 | Tr | 6 |
| Cheese fries with chili | 1 svg | 815 | 44 | 77 | 3 | 29 |
| Cheese fries, smothered | 1 svg | 765 | 48 | 69 | 3 | 27 |
| Chicken burger sandwich | 1 | 630 | 32 | 53 | 2 | 35 |
| Chicken burger buffalo sandwich | 1 | 800 | 45 | 67 | 2 | 37 |
| Chicken fried steak | 4 oz | 265 | 17 | 14 | 1 | 15 |
| Chicken strips, 5 per svg | 1 svg | 720 | 33 | 56 | 2 | 47 |
| Chicken strips buffalo, 5 per svg | 1 svg | 735 | 42 | 43 | 1 | 48 |
| Chili with cheese topping | 1 svg | 400 | 19 | 21 | 1 | 26 |
| Chocolate layer cake | 1 slice | 275 | 12 | 42 | 2 | 4 |
| Club sandwich | 1 | 720 | 38 | 62 | 2 | 32 |
| Corn with butter sauce | 1 svg | 120 | 4 | 19 | 2 | 3 |

78

| FAST FOOD RESTAURANT: (See other Foods and Beverages listed separately) | Serv-ing Size | Cal-ories | Fat (g) | Carb (g) | Fi-ber (g) | Pro-tein (g) |
|---|---|---|---|---|---|---|
| Country fried potatoes | 1 svg | 515 | 35 | 23 | 3 | 3 |
| Double scoop sundae | 1 | 375 | 27 | 29 | 1 | 6 |
| French fries | 1 svg | 260 | 12 | 35 | 3 | 5 |
| French fries w/ seasoning | 1 svg | 320 | 14 | 44 | 4 | 5 |
| Fried shrimp dinner | 8 oz | 220 | 10 | 18 | 1 | 17 |
| Garden salad deluxe w/ chicken | 1 | 265 | 11 | 10 | 5 | 32 |
| Grasshopper blender blaster | 15 oz | 735 | 37 | 92 | 1 | 13 |
| Grasshopper sundae | 14 oz | 735 | 34 | 97 | 1 | 13 |
| Green beans w/ bacon | 1 svg | 60 | 4 | 6 | 2 | 1 |
| Green peas w/ butter sauce | 1 svg | 100 | 2 | 14 | 3 | 5 |
| Grilled chicken dinner | 1 | 130 | 4 | 0 | 0 | 24 |
| Grilled chicken sandwich | 1 | 435 | 9 | 56 | 2 | 35 |
| Grilled chicken stir fried | 1 | 865 | 10 | 149 | 3 | 43 |
| Grilled salmon dinner | 6 oz | 210 | 4 | 1 | 0 | 43 |
| Ham & Swiss sandwich | 1 | 535 | 31 | 40 | 2 | 23 |
| Hamburger, bacon & cheddar | 1 | 875 | 52 | 58 | 2 | 53 |
| Hamburger, big Texas BBQ | 1 | 930 | 58 | 53 | 2 | 53 |
| Hamburger, boca | 1 | 615 | 28 | 66 | 2 | 29 |
| Hamburger, classic | 1 | 675 | 40 | 42 | 2 | 37 |
| Hamburger, classic doubledecker | 1 | 1375 | 92 | 81 | 3 | 62 |
| Hamburger, classic w/ cheese | 1 | 836 | 53 | 43 | 2 | 47 |
| Hamburger, mushroom & Swiss | 1 | 872 | 51 | 58 | 2 | 48 |
| Hot fudge cake sundae | 1 svg | 620 | 35 | 73 | 2 | 7 |
| Malted milk shake, chocolate | 12 oz | 585 | 26 | 82 | 1 | 12 |
| Malted milk shake, vanilla | 12 oz | 585 | 26 | 82 | Tr | 12 |
| Mashed potatoes | 1 svg | 105 | 1 | 21 | 2 | 3 |
| Mashed potatoes w/ cheddar | 1 svg | 117 | 2 | 22 | 2 | 3 |
| Mozzarella sticks, 8 per svg | 1 svg | 710 | 41 | 49 | 1 | 36 |
| Onion rings | 1 svg | 380 | 23 | 38 | 2 | 5 |
| Peaches and cream sundae | 1 | 570 | 22 | 91 | 1 | 5 |
| Pie, apple | 1 slice | 475 | 24 | 64 | 2 | 3 |
| Pie, cherry | 1 slice | 630 | 25 | 101 | 3 | 3 |
| Pie, chocolate peanut butter | 1 slice | 655 | 39 | 64 | 3 | 15 |
| Pie, Hershey's chocolate chip | 1 slice | 600 | 36 | 58 | 2 | 6 |
| Pie, Oreo cookies & cream | 1 slice | 650 | 40 | 67 | 2 | 6 |
| Pot roast dinner | 1 | 295 | 11 | 5 | Tr | 42 |
| Roast turkey dinner | 1 | 388 | 3 | 38 | 1 | 46 |
| Reuben sandwich | 1 | 580 | 35 | 37 | 2 | 27 |
| Shake, chocolate | 12 oz | 560 | 26 | 76 | 1 | 11 |
| Shake, vanilla | 12 oz | 560 | 26 | 76 | Tr | 11 |
| Shrimp scampi skillet dinner | 1 svg | 290 | 19 | 3 | Tr | 25 |

| FAST FOOD RESTAURANT: (See other Foods and Beverages listed separately) | Serving Size | Calories | Fat (g) | Carb (g) | Fiber (g) | Protein (g) |
|---|---|---|---|---|---|---|
| Sirloin steak dinner | 8 oz | 340 | 28 | 1 | 0 | 18 |
| Slim slam | 12 oz | 495 | 12 | 98 | 1 | 34 |
| Steak and shrimp dinner | 9 oz | 640 | 42 | 31 | 1 | 36 |
| Super bird sandwich | 1 | 620 | 32 | 48 | 2 | 35 |
| T-bone steak dinner | 14 oz | 860 | 65 | 0 | 0 | 65 |
| Two egg breakfast | 1 | 825 | 67 | 1 | 0 | 6 |
| Turkey breast sandwich | 1 | 475 | 26 | 39 | 2 | 23 |
| Vegetable rice pilaf | 1 svg | 85 | 1 | 16 | 2 | 2 |
| Western wings roundup | 20 oz | 1515 | 88 | 89 | 3 | 89 |
| ***Domino's Pizza*** | ... | ... | . | . | . | . |
| (1 slice= 1/8 pizza) | ... | ... | . | . | . | . |
| Medium 12-inch Pizzas | ... | ... | . | . | . | .. |
| Cheese | ... | ... | . | . | . | . |
|   Classic hand-tossed | 1 slice | 185 | 6 | 28 | 1 | 7 |
|   Crunchy thin crust | 1 slice | 135 | 7 | 14 | 1 | 5 |
|   Ultimate deep dish | 1 slice | 240 | 11 | 28 | 2 | 9 |
| Beef | ... | ... | . | . | . | . |
|   Classic hand-tossed | 1 slice | 225 | 9 | 28 | 2 | 9 |
|   Crunchy thin crust | 1 slice | 175 | 11 | 14 | 1 | 7 |
|   Ultimate deep dish | 1 slice | 277 | 15 | 28 | 2 | 11 |
| Green pepper, mushroom, onion | ... | ... | . | . | . | . |
|   Classic hand-tossed | 1 slice | 190 | 6 | 29 | 2 | 8 |
|   Crunchy thin crust | 1 slice | 142 | 8 | 15 | 1 | 6 |
|   Ultimate deep dish | 1 slice | 244 | 11 | 30 | 2 | 9 |
| Ham | ... | ... | . | . | . | . |
|   Classic hand-tossed | 1 slice | 195 | 6 | 28 | 1 | 9 |
|   Crunchy thin crust | 1 slice | 150 | 8 | 14 | 1 | 7 |
|   Ultimate deep dish | 1 slice | 250 | 12 | 28 | 2 | 11 |
| Ham & pineapple | ... | ... | . | . | . | . |
|   Classic hand-tossed | 1 slice | 200 | 6 | 29 | 2 | 9 |
|   Crunchy thin crust | 1 slice | 150 | 8 | 15 | 1 | 7 |
|   Ultimate deep dish | 1 slice | 250 | 12 | 30 | 2 | 10 |
| Pepperoni | ... | ... | . | . | . | . |
|   Classic hand-tossed | 1 slice | 223 | 9 | 28 | 2 | 9 |
|   Crunchy thin crust | 1 slice | 175 | 11 | 14 | 1 | 7 |
|   Ultimate deep dish | 1 slice | 275 | 14 | 28 | 2 | 11 |
| Pepperoni & sausage | ... | ... | . | . | . | . |
|   Classic hand-tossed | 1 slice | 255 | 12 | 28 | 2 | 10 |
|   Crunchy thin crust | 1 slice | 206 | 14 | 14 | 1 | 8 |
|   Ultimate deep dish | 1 slice | 307 | 17 | 29 | 2 | 12 |
| Sausage | ... | ... | . | . | . | . |

| FAST FOOD RESTAURANT: (See other Foods and Beverages listed separately) | Serv-ing Size | Cal-ories | Fat (g) | Carb (g) | Fi-ber (g) | Pro-tein (g) |
|---|---|---|---|---|---|---|
| Classic hand-tossed | 1 slice | 230 | 10 | 28 | 2 | 9 |
| Crunchy thin crust | 1 slice | 181 | 11 | 14 | 1 | 7 |
| Ultimate deep dish | 1 slice | 283 | 15 | 29 | 2 | 11 |
| Large 14-inch Pizzas | … | … | . | . | . | . |
| Cheese | … | … | . | . | . | . |
| Classic hand-tossed | 1 slice | 256 | 8 | 38 | 2 | 10 |
| Crunchy thin crust | 1 slice | 190 | 10 | 19 | 1 | 7 |
| Ultimate deep dish | 1 slice | 336 | 15 | 41 | 2 | 13 |
| Beef | … | … | . | . | . | . |
| Classic hand-tossed | 1 slice | 310 | 13 | 38 | 2 | 13 |
| Crunchy thin crust | 1 slice | 243 | 15 | 19 | 1 | 10 |
| Ultimate deep dish | 1 slice | 390 | 20 | 41 | 2 | 15 |
| Green pepper, mushroom, onion | … | … | . | . | . | . |
| Classic hand-tossed | 1 slice | 263 | 8 | 39 | 2 | 11 |
| Crunchy thin crust | 1 slice | 200 | 10 | 21 | 2 | 8 |
| Ultimate deep dish | 1 slice | 343 | 15 | 42 | 3 | 13 |
| Ham | … | … | . | . | . | . |
| Classic hand-tossed | 1 slice | 270 | 9 | 38 | 2 | 12 |
| Crunchy thin crust | 1 slice | 204 | 11 | 19 | 1 | 9 |
| Ultimate deep dish | 1 slice | 350 | 16 | 41 | 2 | 15 |
| Ham & pineapple | … | … | . | . | . | . |
| Classic hand-tossed | 1 slice | 275 | 9 | 40 | 2 | 12 |
| Crunchy thin crust | 1 slice | 207 | 11 | 21 | 1 | 9 |
| Ultimate deep dish | 1 slice | 355 | 16 | 42 | 2 | 14 |
| Pepperoni | … | … | . | . | . | . |
| Classic hand-tossed | 1 slice | 305 | 12 | 38 | 2 | 12 |
| Crunchy thin crust | 1 slice | 237 | 15 | 19 | 1 | 10 |
| Ultimate deep dish | 1 slice | 385 | 20 | 41 | 2 | 15 |
| Pepperoni & sausage | … | … | . | . | . | . |
| Classic hand-tossed | 1 slice | 350 | 16 | 39 | 2 | 14 |
| Crunchy thin crust | 1 slice | 282 | 19 | 19 | 2 | 11 |
| Ultimate deep dish | 1 slice | 430 | 23 | 41 | 3 | 17 |
| Sausage | … | … | . | . | . | . |
| Classic hand-tossed | 1 slice | 320 | 14 | 39 | 2 | 13 |
| Crunchy thin crust | 1 slice | 250 | 16 | 20 | 2 | 10 |
| Ultimate deep dish | 1 slice | 400 | 21 | 42 | 3 | 15 |
| Side Orders & Condiments | … | … | . | . | . | . |
| Barbecue buffalo wings | 1 piece | 50 | 3 | 2 | 0 | 6 |
| Blue cheese dipping sauce | 1 svg | 225 | 24 | 2 | 0 | 1 |
| Bread sticks | 1 piece | 115 | 6 | 12 | 0 | 2 |
| Buffalo chicken kickers | 1 piece | 47 | 2 | 3 | 0 | 4 |

| FAST FOOD RESTAURANT: (See other Foods and Beverages listed separately) | Serving Size | Calories | Fat (g) | Carb (g) | Fiber (g) | Protein (g) |
|---|---|---|---|---|---|---|
| Cheesy bread | 1 piece | 125 | 7 | 13 | 0 | 4 |
| Cinnamon stix | 1 piece | 125 | 6 | 15 | 1 | 2 |
| Garlic sauce | 1 svg | 440 | 49 | 0 | 0 | 0 |
| Hot buffalo wings | 1 piece | 45 | 3 | 1 | 0 | 5 |
| Hot dipping sauce | 1 svg | 15 | 0 | 4 | 0 | 0 |
| Marinara dipping sauce | 1 svg | 25 | Tr | 5 | 0 | 1 |
| Ranch dipping sauce | 1 svg | 195 | 21 | 2 | 0 | 1 |
| Sweet icing | 1 svg | 250 | 3 | 57 | 0 | 0 |
| **Dunkin' Donuts** | ... | ... | . | . | . | . |
| Bagels | ... | ... | . | ... | ... | . |
| Berry berry | 1 | 345 | 3 | 69 | 4 | 11 |
| Blueberry | 1 | 350 | 3 | 69 | 4 | 11 |
| Cinnamon raisin | 1 | 335 | 3 | 65 | 3 | 10 |
| Everything | 1 | 430 | 7 | 75 | 3 | 17 |
| Garlic | 1 | 410 | 4 | 79 | 3 | 16 |
| Onion | 1 | 375 | 4 | 71 | 4 | 14 |
| Plain | 1 | 360 | 3 | 69 | 2 | 14 |
| Poppyseed | 1 | 440 | 10 | 72 | 3 | 17 |
| Salt | 1 | 360 | 3 | 69 | 2 | 14 |
| Sesame | 1 | 455 | 11 | 71 | 3 | 18 |
| Sourdough | 1 | 340 | 3 | 65 | 2 | 15 |
| Wheat | 1 | 350 | 5 | 66 | 4 | 13 |
| Cream cheese | ... | ... | . | ... | . | . |
| Chive | 2 oz | 170 | 17 | 4 | 2 | 4 |
| Garden vegetable | 2 oz | 170 | 15 | 4 | 0 | 2 |
| Light | 2 oz | 110 | 9 | 6 | 0 | 4 |
| Plain | 2 oz | 190 | 17 | 4 | 0 | 4 |
| Salmon | 2 oz | 170 | 17 | 2 | 0 | 4 |
| Shedd's buttermatch blend | 1 Tbsp | 80 | 9 | 0 | 0 | 0 |
| Strawberry | 2 oz | 195 | 17 | 9 | 0 | 4 |
| Cookies | ... | ... | . | ... | . | . |
| Chocolate chunk | 1 | 220 | 11 | 28 | 1 | 3 |
| Chocolate chunk w/ walnuts | 1 | 230 | 12 | 27 | 1 | 3 |
| Oatmeal raisin pecan | 1 | 220 | 10 | 29 | 1 | 3 |
| White chocolate chunk | 1 | 235 | 12 | 28 | 1 | 3 |
| Danish | ... | ... | . | ... | . | . |
| Apple | 1 | 250 | 10 | 36 | 0 | 4 |
| Cheese | 1 | 275 | 14 | 32 | 0 | 4 |
| Strawberry cheese | 1 | 250 | 12 | 33 | 0 | 4 |
| Donuts | ... | ... | . | ... | . | . |
| Apple crumb | 1 | 235 | 10 | 34 | 1 | 3 |

| FAST FOOD RESTAURANT: (See other Foods and Beverages listed separately) | Serv-ing Size | Cal-ories | Fat (g) | Carb (g) | Fi-ber (g) | Pro-tein (g) |
|---|---|---|---|---|---|---|
| Apple & spice | 1 | 200 | 8 | 29 | 1 | 3 |
| Bavarian kreme | 1 | 210 | 9 | 30 | 1 | 3 |
| Black raspberry | 1 | 210 | 8 | 32 | 1 | 3 |
| Blueberry cake | 1 | 290 | 16 | 35 | 1 | 3 |
| Blueberry crumb | 1 | 240 | 10 | 36 | 1 | 3 |
| Boston kreme | 1 | 240 | 9 | 36 | 1 | 3 |
| Chocolate coconut cake | 1 | 300 | 19 | 31 | 1 | 4 |
| Chocolate frosted cake | 1 | 360 | 20 | 40 | 1 | 4 |
| Chocolate frosted | 1 | 200 | 9 | 29 | 1 | 3 |
| Chocolate glazed cake | 1 | 295 | 16 | 33 | 1 | 3 |
| Chocolate kreme filled | 1 | 270 | 13 | 35 | 1 | 3 |
| Cinnamon cake | 1 | 330 | 20 | 34 | 1 | 4 |
| Double chocolate cake | 1 | 310 | 17 | 39 | 2 | 3 |
| French cruller | 1 | 150 | 18 | 17 | 1 | 2 |
| Glazed cake | 1 | 350 | 19 | 41 | 1 | 4 |
| Glazed | 1 | 180 | 8 | 25 | 1 | 3 |
| Jelly filled | 1 | 210 | 8 | 32 | 1 | 3 |
| Maple frosted | 1 | 210 | 9 | 30 | 1 | 3 |
| Marble frosted | 1 | 200 | 9 | 29 | 1 | 3 |
| Old fashioned cake | 1 | 300 | 19 | 28 | 1 | 4 |
| Powdered cake | 1 | 330 | 19 | 36 | 1 | 4 |
| Strawberry | 1 | 210 | 8 | 32 | 1 | 3 |
| Strawberry frosted | 1 | 210 | 9 | 30 | 1 | 3 |
| Sugar raised | 1 | 170 | 8 | 22 | 1 | 3 |
| Vanilla kreme filled | 1 | 170 | 13 | 36 | 1 | 3 |
| Whole white glazed cake | 1 | 310 | 19 | 32 | 1 | 4 |
| Donut-Fancies | … | … | . | . | . | . |
| Apple fritter | 1 | 300 | 14 | 41 | 1 | 4 |
| Bow tie donut | 1 | 300 | 17 | 34 | 1 | 4 |
| Chocolate frosted coffee roll | 1 | 290 | 15 | 36 | 1 | 4 |
| Chocolate iced Bismarck | 1 | 340 | 15 | 50 | 1 | 3 |
| Coffee roll | 1 | 270 | 14 | 33 | 1 | 4 |
| Éclair | 1 | 270 | 11 | 39 | 1 | 3 |
| Glazed fritter | 1 | 260 | 14 | 31 | 1 | 4 |
| Maple frosted coffee roll | 1 | 290 | 14 | 36 | 1 | 4 |
| Vanilla frosted coffee roll | 1 | 290 | 14 | 36 | 1 | 4 |
| Donut-Munchkins | … | … | . | . | . | . |
| Cinnamon cake | 4 | 275 | 15 | 31 | 1 | 3 |
| Glazed | 5 | 200 | 9 | 27 | 1 | 3 |
| Glazed cake | 3 | 280 | 13 | 38 | 1 | 3 |
| Glazed chocolate cake | 3 | 200 | 10 | 26 | 1 | 2 |

| FAST FOOD RESTAURANT: (See other Foods and Beverages listed separately) | Serv-ing Size | Cal-ories | Fat (g) | Carb (g) | Fi-ber (g) | Pro-tein (g) |
|---|---|---|---|---|---|---|
| Jelly filled | 5 | 210 | 9 | 30 | 1 | 3 |
| Lemon filled | 4 | 170 | 8 | 23 | 0 | 2 |
| Plain cake | 4 | 270 | 16 | 27 | 1 | 3 |
| Powdered cake | 4 | 270 | 14 | 31 | 1 | 3 |
| Sugar raised | 7 | 220 | 12 | 26 | 1 | 4 |
| Donut-Sticks | ... | ... | . | . | . | . |
| Cinnamon cake | 1 | 450 | 30 | 42 | 1 | 4 |
| Glazed cake | 1 | 490 | 29 | 51 | 1 | 4 |
| Glazed chocolate cake | 1 | 470 | 29 | 49 | 2 | 4 |
| Jelly | 1 | 530 | 29 | 61 | 1 | 4 |
| Plain cake | 1 | 420 | 29 | 35 | 1 | 4 |
| Powdered cake | 1 | 450 | 29 | 42 | 1 | 4 |
| Muffins | ... | ... | . | . | . | . |
| Banana walnut | 1 | 545 | 23 | 73 | 3 | 10 |
| Blueberry | 1 | 490 | 18 | 75 | 2 | 8 |
| Carrot walnut spice | 1 | 600 | 27 | 81 | 3 | 8 |
| Chocolate chip | 1 | 590 | 23 | 85 | 3 | 9 |
| Coffee cake with topping | 1 | 710 | 29 | 102 | 2 | 11 |
| Corn | 1 | 510 | 17 | 81 | 1 | 9 |
| Cranberry orange | 1 | 460 | 16 | 71 | 3 | 8 |
| Honey bran raisin | 1 | 490 | 14 | 81 | 5 | 10 |
| Reduced fat blueberry | 1 | 450 | 13 | 74 | 2 | 9 |
| Other Misc. Items | ... | ... | . | ... | . | . |
| Apple pie | 1 svg | 615 | 28 | 82 | 4 | 9 |
| Apple pie a la mode | 1 svg | 810 | 38 | 107 | 4 | 12 |
| Biscuit, plain | 1 | 250 | 13 | 29 | 1 | 5 |
| Croissant, plain | 1 | 330 | 18 | 37 | 0 | 5 |
| Scone, maple walnut | 1 | 470 | 22 | 62 | 1 | 6 |
| Scone, raspberry white choc. | 1 | 450 | 22 | 59 | 2 | 6 |
| Sandwiches, Breakfast type | ... | ... | . | . | . | . |
| Bagel w/ egg, bacon, cheese | 1 | 500 | 13 | 71 | 2 | 26 |
| Bagel w/ egg, ham, cheese | 1 | 500 | 11 | 70 | 2 | 29 |
| Bagel w/ egg, sausage, cheese | 1 | 675 | 28 | 71 | 2 | 32 |
| Biscuit w/ egg & cheese | 1 | 360 | 20 | 31 | 1 | 14 |
| Biscuit w/ sausage, egg, cheese | 1 | 560 | 38 | 31 | 1 | 23 |
| Croissant w/ egg, ham, cheese | 1 | 470 | 27 | 38 | 0 | 20 |
| English muffin w/egg, cheese | 1 | 270 | 8 | 35 | 1 | 15 |
| English muffin w/ egg, bacon & cheese | ...<br>1 | ...<br>310 | .<br>11 | .<br>35 | .<br>1 | .<br>18 |
| English muffin w/ egg, ham, & cheese | ...<br>1 | ...<br>310 | .<br>10 | .<br>35 | .<br>1 | .<br>21 |

| FAST FOOD RESTAURANT: (See other Foods and Beverages listed separately) | Serv-ing Size | Cal-ories | Fat (g) | Carb (g) | Fi-ber (g) | Pro-tein (g) |
|---|---|---|---|---|---|---|
| Beverages | ... | ... | . | . | . | . |
| Cappuccino | 10 oz | 80 | 5 | 7 | 0 | 4 |
| Cappuccino with sugar | 10 oz | 130 | 5 | 21 | 0 | 4 |
| Coffee | 10 oz | 15 | 0 | 3 | 0 | 1 |
| Coffee with cream | 10 oz | 70 | 6 | 3 | 0 | 1 |
| Coffee with cream and sugar | 10 oz | 120 | 6 | 15 | 0 | 1 |
| Coffee with milk | 10 oz | 35 | 1 | 4 | 0 | 2 |
| Coffee with milk and sugar | 10 oz | 80 | 1 | 16 | 0 | 2 |
| Coffee with skim milk | 10 oz | 25 | 0 | 4 | 0 | 2 |
| Coffee w/ skim milk & sugar | 10 oz | 70 | 0 | 16 | 0 | 2 |
| Coffee with sugar | 10 oz | 60 | 0 | 15 | 0 | 1 |
| Coffee coolatta with 2% milk | 16 oz | 190 | 2 | 41 | 0 | 4 |
| Coffee coolatta with cream | 16 oz | 350 | 22 | 40 | 0 | 3 |
| Coffee coolatta with milk | 16 oz | 210 | 4 | 42 | 0 | 4 |
| Coffee coolatta w/skim milk | 16 oz | 170 | 0 | 41 | 0 | 4 |
| Coolatta, strawberry fruit | 16 oz | 290 | 0 | 72 | 1 | 0 |
| Coolatta, vanilla bean | 16 oz | 440 | 17 | 70 | 1 | 1 |
| Dunkaccino | 10 oz | 230 | 10 | 35 | 0 | 2 |
| Espresso | 2 oz | 1 | 0 | 1 | 0 | 0 |
| Espresso with sugar | 2 oz | 30 | 0 | 7 | 0 | 0 |
| Hot chocolate | 10 oz | 220 | 8 | 38 | 2 | 2 |
| Latte, plain | 10 oz | 120 | 6 | 10 | 0 | 6 |
| Latte with sugar | 10 oz | 160 | 6 | 22 | 0 | 6 |
| Latte w/ Caramel swirl | 10 oz | 230 | 6 | 36 | 0 | 8 |
| Latte w/ Mocha swirl | 10 oz | 230 | 7 | 37 | 1 | 6 |
| Iced coffee | 16 oz | 15 | 0 | 3 | 0 | 1 |
| Iced coffee with cream | 16 oz | 70 | 6 | 4 | 0 | 2 |
| Iced coffee w/cream & sugar | 16 oz | 120 | 6 | 16 | 0 | 2 |
| Iced coffee with milk | 16 oz | 35 | 1 | 4 | 0 | 2 |
| Iced coffee w/ milk and sugar | 16 oz | 80 | 1 | 16 | 0 | 2 |
| Iced coffee with skim milk | 16 oz | 25 | 0 | 4 | 0 | 2 |
| Iced coffee w/skim milk, sugar | 16 oz | 70 | 0 | 16 | 0 | 2 |
| Iced latte | 16 oz | 120 | 7 | 11 | 0 | 6 |
| Iced latte with sugar | 16 oz | 170 | 7 | 23 | 0 | 6 |
| Iced caramel swirl latte | 16 oz | 240 | 7 | 37 | 0 | 8 |
| Iced mocha swirl latte | 16 oz | 240 | 8 | 38 | 1 | 7 |
| Vanilla chai | 10 oz | 230 | 8 | 40 | 0 | 1 |
| Tea, plain, w/o milk or sugar | ... | ... | . | . | . | . |
| Decaffeinated tea | 10 oz | 0 | 0 | 1 | 0 | 0 |
| Earl Grey tea | 10 oz | 0 | 0 | 1 | 0 | 0 |
| English breakfast tea | 10 oz | 0 | 0 | 1 | 0 | 0 |

| FAST FOOD RESTAURANT: (See other Foods and Beverages listed separately) | Serving Size | Calories | Fat (g) | Carb (g) | Fiber (g) | Protein (g) |
|---|---|---|---|---|---|---|
| Green tea | 10 oz | 0 | 0 | 1 | 0 | 0 |
| Regular tea | 10 oz | 0 | 0 | 1 | 0 | 0 |
| Regular tea w/ lemon | 10 oz | 0 | 0 | 1 | 0 | 0 |
| Tea w/ regular milk, no sugar | 10 oz | 25 | 1 | 2 | 0 | 1 |
| Tea w/ regular milk and sugar | 10 oz | 70 | 1 | 14 | 0 | 1 |
| Tea w/ skim milk, no sugar | 10 oz | 25 | Tr | 4 | 0 | 1 |
| Tea w/ skim milk and sugar | 10 oz | 60 | Tr | 14 | 0 | 1 |
| **Hardees** | ... | ... | . | . | . | . |
| Apple cinnamon raisin biscuit | 1 | 200 | 8 | 30 | 2 | 2 |
| Bacon & egg biscuit | 1 | 575 | 33 | 45 | 2 | 22 |
| Bacon, egg & cheese biscuit | 1 | 610 | 37 | 45 | 2 | 24 |
| Baked beans | 1 svg | 170 | 1 | 32 | 4 | 8 |
| Big chocolate chip cookie | 1 | 280 | 12 | 41 | 2 | 4 |
| Big country bacon | 1 svg | 820 | 49 | 62 | 2 | 33 |
| Big country sausage | 1 svg | 995 | 66 | 62 | 2 | 41 |
| Big roast beef | 1 | 465 | 24 | 35 | 3 | 26 |
| Biscuits w/ gravy | 1 svg | 495 | 28 | 55 | 3 | 10 |
| Cheeseburger | 1 | 310 | 14 | 30 | 2 | 16 |
| Chicken, breast | 1 piece | 370 | 15 | 29 | 2 | 29 |
| Chicken, leg | 1 piece | 170 | 7 | 15 | 1 | 13 |
| Chicken, thigh | 1 piece | 330 | 15 | 30 | 2 | 39 |
| Chicken, wing | 1 piece | 195 | 8 | 23 | 1 | 10 |
| Chicken fillet sandwich | 1 | 480 | 18 | 54 | 3 | 26 |
| Chocolate cone | 1 | 180 | 3 | 34 | 1 | 5 |
| Chocolate shake | 1 | 375 | 5 | 67 | 1 | 13 |
| Cole slaw | 1 svg | 240 | 20 | 13 | 3 | 2 |
| Cool twist cone | 1 | 180 | 2 | 34 | 1 | 4 |
| Country ham biscuit | 1 | 430 | 22 | 45 | 3 | 15 |
| Cravin bacon cheeseburger | 1 | 690 | 46 | 38 | 2 | 30 |
| Fat free French dressing | 1 svg | 70 | 0 | 17 | Tr | 0 |
| Fisherman's fillet | 1 | 565 | 27 | 54 | 3 | 26 |
| French fries, large | 1 | 430 | 18 | 59 | 4 | 6 |
| French fries, medium | 1 | 350 | 15 | 49 | 3 | 5 |
| French fries, small | 1 | 240 | 10 | 33 | 2 | 4 |
| Frisco ham sandwich | 1 | 500 | 25 | 46 | 3 | 24 |
| Frisco sandwich | 1 | 720 | 46 | 43 | 3 | 33 |
| Garden salad | 1 | 220 | 13 | 11 | 3 | 12 |
| Gravy, 1.5 oz | 1 svg | 22 | 1 | 3 | Tr | 1 |
| Grilled chicken | 1 | 350 | 11 | 38 | 2 | 25 |
| Chilled chicken salad | 1 | 150 | 3 | 11 | 3 | 20 |
| Ham biscuit | 1 | 400 | 30 | 47 | 3 | 9 |

| FAST FOOD RESTAURANT: (See other Foods and Beverages listed separately) | Serv- ing Size | Cal- ories | Fat (g) | Carb (g) | Fi- ber (g) | Pro- tein (g) |
|---|---|---|---|---|---|---|
| Ham, egg, & cheese biscuit | 1 | 540 | 30 | 48 | 3 | 20 |
| Hamburger | 1 | 270 | 11 | 29 | 2 | 14 |
| Hot fudge sundae | 1 | 180 | 6 | 51 | 1 | 7 |
| Hot ham & cheese | 1 | 310 | 12 | 34 | 2 | 16 |
| Jelly biscuit | 1 | 440 | 21 | 57 | 3 | 6 |
| Mashed potatoes | 1 svg | 70 | 1 | 14 | 3 | 2 |
| Mesquite bacon cheeseburger | 1 | 370 | 18 | 32 | 2 | 19 |
| Mushroom & Swiss burger | 1 | 490 | 25 | 39 | 2 | 28 |
| Pancakes, 3 per svg | 1 svg | 280 | 2 | 56 | 3 | 8 |
| Peach cobbler | 1 svg | 310 | 7 | 60 | 2 | 2 |
| Peach shake | 1 | 390 | 4 | 77 | 1 | 10 |
| Quarter Lb double cheeseburger | 1 | 470 | 27 | 31 | 3 | 27 |
| Ranch dressing | 1 svg | 290 | 29 | 6 | Tr | 1 |
| Regular hash rounds | 1 svg | 230 | 14 | 24 | 2 | 3 |
| Regular roast beef | 1 | 320 | 16 | 26 | 2 | 17 |
| Rise & shine biscuit | 1 | 390 | 21 | 44 | 2 | 6 |
| Sausage biscuit | 1 | 510 | 31 | 44 | 2 | 14 |
| Sausage & egg biscuit | 1 | 630 | 40 | 45 | 2 | 23 |
| Side salad, w/o dressing | 1 | 25 | Tr | 4 | 2 | 1 |
| Strawberry shake | 1 | 420 | 4 | 83 | 1 | 11 |
| Strawberry sundae | 1 | 210 | 2 | 43 | 1 | 5 |
| The boss | 1 | 570 | 33 | 42 | 3 | 27 |
| The works burger | 1 | 530 | 30 | 41 | 3 | 25 |
| Thousand island dressing | 1 svg | 250 | 23 | 9 | Tr | 1 |
| Ultimate omelet biscuit | 1 | 570 | 33 | 45 | 2 | 22 |
| Vanilla cone | 1 | 170 | 2 | 34 | 1 | 4 |
| Vanilla shake | 1 | 350 | 5 | 65 | 1 | 12 |
| **Jack-In-The-Box** | ... | ... | . | . | . | . |
| Breakfast Jack | 1 | 295 | 12 | 30 | 1 | 18 |
| Breakfast sandwich, sourdough | 1 | 380 | 20 | 31 | 2 | 21 |
| Carrot cake | 1 piece | 365 | 15 | 58 | 2 | 3 |
| Cheeseburger, regular | 1 | 320 | 15 | 32 | 2 | 16 |
| Cheeseburger, double | 1 | 450 | 24 | 35 | 2 | 24 |
| Cheeseburger, ultimate | 1 | 1025 | 79 | 30 | 3 | 50 |
| Cheesecake | 1 piece | 310 | 18 | 29 | 1 | 8 |
| Chicken pita fajita | 1 | 290 | 8 | 29 | 2 | 24 |
| Chicken sandwich, regular | 1 | 400 | 18 | 38 | 2 | 20 |
| Chicken sandwich, Caesar | 1 | 520 | 26 | 44 | 2 | 27 |
| Chicken sandwich, grilled | 1 | 430 | 19 | 36 | 2 | 29 |
| Chicken sandwich, spicy | 1 | 560 | 27 | 55 | 2 | 24 |
| Chicken sandwich, super | 1 | 615 | 36 | 48 | 2 | 25 |

| FAST FOOD RESTAURANT: (See other Foods and Beverages listed separately) | Serv- ing Size | Cal- ories | Fat (g) | Carb (g) | Fi- ber (g) | Pro- tein (g) |
|---|---|---|---|---|---|---|
| Chicken strips, 6 per svg | 1 svg | 450 | 20 | 28 | 1 | 39 |
| Chicken teriyaki | 1 svg | 580 | 2 | 115 | 5 | 28 |
| Egg roll | 1 piece | 150 | 8 | 18 | 1 | 1 |
| Egg rolls, 5 piece serving | 5 piece | 745 | 41 | 92 | 3 | 5 |
| French fries, curly | 1 | 360 | 20 | 39 | 3 | 5 |
| French fries, jumbo size | 1 | 400 | 19 | 51 | 3 | 5 |
| French fries, regular size | 1 | 350 | 17 | 45 | 3 | 4 |
| French fries, small | 1 | 220 | 11 | 28 | 2 | 3 |
| French fries, super size | 1 | 590 | 29 | 76 | 5 | 8 |
| Hamburger | 1 | 280 | 11 | 31 | 2 | 13 |
| Hash browns | 2 oz | 160 | 11 | 14 | 2 | 1 |
| Jalapenos, stuffed | 1 svg | 600 | 39 | 41 | 2 | 22 |
| Jumbo Jack | 1 | 560 | 32 | 41 | 2 | 26 |
| Jumbo Jack w/ cheese | 1 | 650 | 40 | 42 | 2 | 31 |
| Onion rings | 1 svg | 380 | 23 | 38 | 2 | 5 |
| Pancake platter | 1 svg | 400 | 12 | 59 | 3 | 13 |
| Potato wedges, bacon & cheddar | 1 svg | 795 | 58 | 49 | 4 | 20 |
| Sausage croissant | 1 | 675 | 48 | 39 | 2 | 21 |
| Scrambled egg pocket | 1 | 430 | 21 | 31 | 1 | 29 |
| Shake, cappuccino | 1 large | 625 | 28 | 80 | 1 | 11 |
| Shake, chocolate | 1 large | 625 | 27 | 85 | 1 | 11 |
| Shake, strawberry | 1 large | 630 | 28 | 85 | 1 | 10 |
| Shake, vanilla | 1 large | 615 | 30 | 73 | 0 | 12 |
| Supreme croissant | 1 | 570 | 36 | 39 | 2 | 21 |
| Taco | 1 | 185 | 11 | 15 | 2 | 7 |
| Taco monster | 1 | 285 | 17 | 22 | 3 | 12 |
| **Kentucky Fried Chicken** | ... | ... | . | . | . | . |
| Barbecue baked beans | 1 svg | 185 | 3 | 33 | 6 | 6 |
| Biscuit | 1 | 180 | 10 | 20 | 2 | 4 |
| Breast, extra tasty crispy | 1 | 470 | 28 | 25 | 1 | 31 |
| Breast, hot & spicy | 1 | 520 | 34 | 23 | 1 | 32 |
| Breast, original recipe | 1 | 400 | 25 | 16 | 1 | 29 |
| Breast, tender roast | 1 | 255 | 24 | 1 | Tr | 29 |
| Chunky chicken pot pie | 1 | 775 | 42 | 69 | 4 | 29 |
| Coleslaw | 5 oz | 180 | 9 | 21 | 4 | 2 |
| Cornbread | 1 piece | 228 | 13 | 18 | 3 | 27 |
| Corn on the cob | 1 | 190 | 3 | 34 | 4 | 5 |
| Crispy strips, 3 pieces/svg | 1 svg | 260 | 16 | 10 | 3 | 20 |
| Drumstick, original recipe | 1 | 160 | 9 | 6 | 1 | 15 |
| Drumstick, tender roast | 1 | 100 | 4 | 1 | 0 | 13 |
| Green beans | 1 svg | 45 | 5 | 7 | 3 | 1 |

| FAST FOOD RESTAURANT: (See other Foods and Beverages listed separately) | Serv-ing Size | Cal-ories | Fat (g) | Carb (g) | Fi-ber (g) | Pro-tein (g) |
|---|---|---|---|---|---|---|
| Hot wings, 6 pieces/svg | 1 svg | 470 | 33 | 18 | 2 | 27 |
| Kentucky nuggets , 6 pieces/svg | 1 svg | 285 | 18 | 15 | 1 | 16 |
| Macaroni and cheese | med | 180 | 8 | 21 | 3 | 7 |
| Original recipe chicken | … | … | . | . | . | . |
| sandwich | 1 | 495 | 22 | 46 | 3 | 29 |
| Potato salad | 1 svg | 230 | 14 | 23 | 3 | 4 |
| Potato wedges | 1 svg | 280 | 13 | 28 | 3 | 5 |
| Potatoes, mashed | 1 svg | 120 | 6 | 17 | 3 | 1 |
| Red beans and rice | 1 svg | 130 | 3 | 21 | 3 | 5 |
| Thigh, extra tasty crispy or hot | 1 | 370 | 25 | 18 | 1 | 19 |
| Thigh, original recipe | 1 | 255 | 18 | 6 | 1 | 16 |
| Thigh, tender roast | 1 | 205 | 12 | 1 | 0 | 18 |
| Value BBQ chicken sandwich | 1 | 255 | 8 | 28 | 2 | 17 |
| Wing, extra tasty crispy or hot | 1 | 210 | 15 | 9 | 1 | 10 |
| Wing, original recipe | 1 | 140 | 10 | 5 | Tr | 9 |
| Wing, tender roast | 1 | 121 | 8 | 1 | Tr | 12 |
| **Krispy Kreme Doughnuts** | … | … | . | . | . | . |
| Apple fritter | 1 | 385 | 21 | 46 | Tr | 4 |
| Caramel creme crunch | 1 | 350 | 19 | 43 | Tr | 4 |
| Chocolate iced cake | 1 | 270 | 14 | 36 | Tr | 3 |
| Chocolate iced cake w/ sprinkles | 1 | 290 | 14 | 40 | Tr | 3 |
| Chocolate iced crème filled | 1 | 350 | 21 | 39 | Tr | 3 |
| Chocolate iced cruller | 1 | 290 | 15 | 37 | Tr | 2 |
| Chocolate iced custard filled | 1 | 300 | 17 | 35 | Tr | 3 |
| Chocolate iced glazed | 1 | 250 | 12 | 33 | Tr | 3 |
| Chocolate iced glazed, sprinkles | 1 | 200 | 12 | 38 | Tr | 3 |
| Chocolate malted kreme | 1 | 395 | 21 | 49 | Tr | 4 |
| Cinnamon apple filled | 1 | 290 | 16 | 32 | Tr | 3 |
| Cinnamon bun | 1 | 260 | 16 | 28 | Tr | 3 |
| Cinnamon sugar cake | 1 | 280 | 14 | 37 | Tr | 3 |
| Cinnamon twist | 1 | 230 | 9 | 33 | Tr | 3 |
| Coffee & kreme | 1 | 360 | 20 | 43 | Tr | 3 |
| Dulce de leche | 1 | 295 | 18 | 30 | Tr | 3 |
| Glazed blueberry cake | 1 | 340 | 18 | 42 | Tr | 3 |
| Glazed blueberry filled | 1 | 290 | 16 | 35 | Tr | 3 |
| Glazed cinnamon | 1 | 210 | 12 | 24 | Tr | 2 |
| Glazed crème filled | 1 | 345 | 20 | 39 | Tr | 3 |
| Glazed cruller | 1 | 240 | 14 | 26 | Tr | 2 |
| Glazed custard filled | 1 | 290 | 16 | 34 | Tr | 3 |
| Glazed devil's food cake | 1 | 340 | 18 | 42 | Tr | 3 |
| Glazed lemon filled | 1 | 290 | 16 | 34 | Tr | 3 |

| FAST FOOD RESTAURANT: (See other Foods and Beverages listed separately) | Serv-ing Size | Cal-ories | Fat (g) | Carb (g) | Fi-ber (g) | Pro-tein (g) |
|---|---|---|---|---|---|---|
| Glazed sour cream | 1 | 340 | 18 | 42 | Tr | 3 |
| Glazed raspberry filled | 1 | 300 | 16 | 39 | Tr | 3 |
| Glazed strawberry filled | 1 | 290 | 16 | 35 | Tr | 3 |
| Glazed twist | 1 | 210 | 9 | 28 | Tr | 3 |
| Honey and oat | 1 | 340 | 18 | 42 | Tr | 3 |
| Key lime pie | 1 | 330 | 18 | 40 | Tr | 3 |
| Maple iced | 1 | 240 | 12 | 32 | Tr | 2 |
| Maple iced cake | 1 | 270 | 13 | 35 | Tr | 3 |
| New York cheesecake | 1 | 330 | 19 | 36 | Tr | 4 |
| Original glazed | 1 | 200 | 12 | 22 | Tr | 2 |
| Powdered blueberry filled | 1 | 290 | 16 | 32 | Tr | 3 |
| Powdered cake | 1 | 280 | 14 | 37 | Tr | 3 |
| Powdered crème filled | 1 | 345 | 21 | 36 | Tr | 3 |
| Powdered raspberry | 1 | 300 | 16 | 36 | Tr | 3 |
| Powdered strawberry filled | 1 | 260 | 16 | 26 | Tr | 3 |
| Pumpkin spice cake | 1 | 340 | 18 | 42 | Tr | 3 |
| Sugar coated | 1 | 200 | 12 | 21 | Tr | 2 |
| Traditional cake | 1 | 230 | 13 | 25 | Tr | 3 |
| Vanilla iced cake w/ sprinkles | 1 | 270 | 13 | 35 | Tr | 3 |
| Vanilla iced crème filled | 1 | 345 | 20 | 38 | Tr | 3 |
| Vanilla iced custard filled | 1 | 290 | 16 | 33 | Tr | 3 |
| Vanilla iced glazed | 1 | 240 | 12 | 32 | Tr | 2 |
| Vanilla iced raspberry filled | 1 | 355 | 16 | 50 | Tr | 3 |
| Vanilla iced raspberry glazed | 1 | 355 | 16 | 50 | Tr | 3 |
| **Long John Silver's** | ... | ... | . | . | . | . |
| Cheesesticks, 3 per svg | 1 svg | 165 | 9 | 12 | 1 | 6 |
| Chicken, battered plank | 1 | 145 | 8 | 9 | 1 | 8 |
| Chicken sandwich | 1 | 340 | 14 | 40 | 2 | 13 |
| Chicken sandwich w/ cheese | 1 | 390 | 19 | 40 | 2 | 16 |
| Clam chowder | 1 svg | 525 | 24 | 52 | 4 | 24 |
| Clams, breaded | 1 svg | 250 | 14 | 26 | 2 | 9 |
| Cole slaw | 4 oz | 170 | 7 | 23 | 5 | 2 |
| Crabcake | 1 | 150 | 9 | 12 | 1 | 4 |
| Fish, battered | 1 piece | 230 | 13 | 16 | 2 | 12 |
| Fish, battered, junior size | 1 piece | 120 | 8 | 8 | 1 | 5 |
| Fish, country breaded | 1 piece | 200 | 10 | 17 | 2 | 10 |
| Fish w/lemon crumb | 2 piece | 240 | 12 | 10 | 2 | 23 |
| Fish sandwich | 1 | 430 | 20 | 46 | 3 | 16 |
| Fish sandwich w/ cheese | 1 | 485 | 25 | 46 | 3 | 19 |
| Fish sandwich, ultimate | 1 | 490 | 26 | 46 | 3 | 19 |
| French fries, regular size | 1 | 250 | 15 | 28 | 2 | 3 |

| FAST FOOD RESTAURANT: (See other Foods and Beverages listed separately) | Serv-ing Size | Cal-ories | Fat (g) | Carb (g) | Fi-ber (g) | Pro-tein (g) |
|---|---|---|---|---|---|---|
| French fries, large size | 1 | 420 | 24 | 46 | 4 | 5 |
| Grilled chicken salad | 1 | 140 | 3 | 20 | 3 | 10 |
| Hushpuppies | 2 piece | 120 | 6 | 50 | 2 | 18 |
| Ocean chef salad | 1 | 128 | 2 | 15 | 3 | 14 |
| Pie, banana split sundae | 1 svg | 300 | 17 | 34 | 2 | 4 |
| Pie, chocolate crème | 1 svg | 285 | 17 | 29 | 3 | 4 |
| Pie, Dutch apple | 1 svg | 290 | 13 | 44 | 3 | 2 |
| Pie, pecan | 1 svg | 390 | 19 | 53 | 3 | 3 |
| Pie, strawberries & cream | 1 svg | 280 | 15 | 32 | 3 | 4 |
| Pineapple crème cheesecake | 1 svg | 310 | 17 | 36 | 3 | 4 |
| Shrimp, battered | 1 piece | 45 | 3 | 3 | 1 | 2 |
| Shrimp, battered, popcorn | 1 svg | 325 | 15 | 33 | 3 | 15 |
| **McDonald's** | ... | ... | . | . | . | . |
| Apple bran muffin, lowfat | 1 | 300 | 3 | 61 | 3 | 6 |
| Apple Danish | 1 | 360 | 16 | 51 | 1 | 5 |
| Apple pie, baked | 1 | 260 | 13 | 34 | 1 | 3 |
| Arch deluxe | 1 | 550 | 31 | 69 | 4 | 28 |
| Arch deluxe with bacon | 1 | 590 | 34 | 38 | 4 | 32 |
| Bacon, egg & cheese biscuit | 1 | 440 | 26 | 33 | 1 | 17 |
| Barbecue sauce | 1 svg | 45 | 0 | 10 | 0 | 0 |
| Big mac | 1 | 560 | 31 | 45 | 3 | 26 |
| Biscuit, plain | 1 | 260 | 13 | 32 | 1 | 4 |
| Breakfast burrito | 1 | 320 | 20 | 23 | 1 | 13 |
| Caesar salad | 1 | 160 | 14 | 7 | 0 | 2 |
| Chef salad | 1 | 230 | 13 | 8 | 3 | 21 |
| Cheese Danish | 1 | 410 | 22 | 47 | 0 | 7 |
| Cheeseburger | 1 | 320 | 13 | 35 | 2 | 15 |
| Chicken McNuggets, 4 pieces | 1 svg | 190 | 11 | 10 | 0 | 12 |
| Chicken McNuggets, 6 pieces | 1 svg | 290 | 17 | 15 | 0 | 18 |
| Chicken McNuggets, 9 pieces | 1 svg | 430 | 26 | 23 | 0 | 27 |
| Chocolate chip cookie | 1 | 170 | 10 | 22 | 1 | 2 |
| Chocolate shake, small | 1 | 360 | 9 | 60 | 1 | 11 |
| Cinnamon roll | 1 | 400 | 20 | 47 | 2 | 7 |
| Crispy chicken deluxe | 1 | 500 | 25 | 43 | 3 | 26 |
| Croutons | 1 svg | 50 | 5 | 7 | 0 | 2 |
| Egg McMuffin | 1 | 290 | 12 | 27 | 1 | 17 |
| English muffin | 1 | 140 | 2 | 25 | 1 | 4 |
| Fat free herb vinegar dressing | 1 svg | 50 | 0 | 11 | 0 | 1 |
| Fish fillet sandwich | 1 | 560 | 28 | 54 | 4 | 23 |
| French fries, large | 1 | 450 | 22 | 57 | 5 | 6 |
| French fries, small | 1 | 210 | 10 | 26 | 2 | 3 |

| FAST FOOD RESTAURANT: (See other Foods and Beverages listed separately) | Serv- ing Size | Cal- ories | Fat (g) | Carb (g) | Fi- ber (g) | Pro- tein (g) |
|---|---|---|---|---|---|---|
| Garden salad | 1 | 35 | 0 | 7 | 2 | 2 |
| Grilled chicken deluxe | 1 | 440 | 20 | 38 | 3 | 27 |
| Grilled chicken salad deluxe | 1 | 120 | 2 | 7 | 2 | 21 |
| Hamburger | 1 | 260 | 9 | 34 | 2 | 13 |
| Hash browns | 1 svg | 130 | 7 | 53 | 2 | 9 |
| Honey dressing | 1 svg | 45 | 0 | 12 | 0 | 0 |
| Honey mustard dressing | 1 svg | 50 | 5 | 3 | 0 | 0 |
| Hot caramel sundae | 1 | 360 | 10 | 61 | 0 | 7 |
| Hot fudge sundae | 1 | 340 | 12 | 52 | 1 | 8 |
| Hot mustard | 1 svg | 60 | 4 | 7 | 0 | 1 |
| Hotcakes, plain | 1 svg | 310 | 7 | 53 | 2 | 9 |
| Hotcakes w/ syrup & margarine | 1 svg | 580 | 16 | 100 | 2 | 9 |
| Mayonnaise, light | 1 svg | 40 | 4 | 0 | 0 | 0 |
| McDonaldland cookie | 1 | 180 | 5 | 32 | 1 | 3 |
| Quarter pounder | 1 | 420 | 21 | 37 | 2 | 23 |
| Quarter pounder with cheese | 1 | 530 | 30 | 38 | 2 | 28 |
| Red French reduced cal dressing | 1 svg | 160 | 8 | 23 | 0 | 0 |
| Sausage (w/o biscuit) | 1 svg | 170 | 16 | 0 | 0 | 6 |
| Sausage biscuit w/ egg | 1 | 505 | 35 | 33 | 1 | 16 |
| Sausage McMuffin | 1 | 360 | 23 | 26 | 1 | 13 |
| Sausage McMuffin with egg | 1 | 440 | 28 | 27 | 1 | 19 |
| Scrambled eggs, 2 per svg | 1 svg | 160 | 11 | 1 | 0 | 13 |
| Strawberry shake, small | 1 | 360 | 9 | 60 | 0 | 11 |
| Strawberry sundae | 1 | 290 | 7 | 50 | 0 | 7 |
| Sweet & sour sauce | 1 svg | 50 | 0 | 11 | 0 | 0 |
| Vanilla cone, reduced fat | 1 | 150 | 5 | 23 | 0 | 4 |
| Vanilla shake, small | 1 | 360 | 9 | 59 | 0 | 11 |
| **Panda Express Chinese Food** | … | … | . | . | . | . |
| Beef dishes | … | … | . | . | . | . |
| Beef with broccoli | 6 oz | 150 | 8 | 8 | 1 | 11 |
| Beef with string beans | 6 oz | 170 | 9 | 11 | 2 | 12 |
| Chicken dishes | … | … | . | . | . | . |
| Black pepper chicken | 6 oz | 180 | 10 | 10 | 2 | 13 |
| Chicken & orange sauce | 6 oz | 480 | 21 | 50 | 2 | 21 |
| Chicken with mushrooms | 6 oz | 130 | 7 | 7 | 2 | 11 |
| Chicken with string beans | 6 oz | 170 | 8 | 12 | 3 | 11 |
| Hot spicy chicken w/ peanuts | 6 oz | 200 | 7 | 17 | 4 | 18 |
| Mandarin chicken | 6 oz | 250 | 9 | 8 | 2 | 34 |
| Potatoes with chicken | 6 oz | 220 | 11 | 17 | 1 | 12 |
| Sweet & sour chicken | 4 oz | 310 | 14 | 28 | 2 | 18 |
| Pork dishes | … | … | . | . | . | . |

92

| FAST FOOD RESTAURANT: (See other Foods and Beverages listed separately) | Serv-ing Size | Cal-ories | Fat (g) | Carb (g) | Fi-ber (g) | Pro-tein (g) |
|---|---|---|---|---|---|---|
| Barbecue pork | 5 oz | 350 | 19 | 13 | Tr | 32 |
| Sweet & sour pork | 4 oz | 410 | 30 | 17 | 3 | 19 |
| Vegetable dishes | … | … | . | . | . | . |
| Mixed vegetables | 6 oz | 70 | 3 | 8 | 3 | 3 |
| String beans w/fried tofu | 6 oz | 180 | 11 | 11 | 3 | 10 |
| Vegetable chow mein | 8 oz | 330 | 11 | 48 | 4 | 10 |
| Rice | … | … | . | . | . | . |
| Fried rice w/vegetables | 8 oz | 390 | 12 | 61 | 2 | 9 |
| Steamed rice | 8 oz | 330 | 1 | 74 | 2 | 7 |
| Appetizers | … | … | . | . | . | . |
| Fried shrimp | 6 piece | 260 | 12 | 26 | Tr | 12 |
| Chicken egg roll | 1 | 190 | 8 | 21 | 3 | 8 |
| Vegetable spring roll | 1 | 80 | 3 | 14 | 1 | 2 |
| Sauces | … | … | . | . | . | . |
| Hot mustard sauce | 1 svg | 18 | 0 | 1 | 0 | 0 |
| Hot sauce | 2 tsp | 10 | 1 | 2 | 0 | 0 |
| Mandarin sauce | 2 oz | 70 | 0 | 16 | 0 | Tr |
| Sweet & sour sauce | 2 oz | 60 | 0 | 15 | 0 | Tr |
| Soy sauce | 1 Tbsp | 16 | 0 | 2 | 0 | 2 |
| **Papa John's Pizza** | … | … | . | . | . | . |
| Original crust pizza, large-14" | … | … | . | . | . | . |
| Cheese | 1 slice | 290 | 10 | 39 | 2 | 12 |
| Pepperoni | 1 slice | 345 | 15 | 39 | 2 | 14 |
| Sausage | 1 slice | 335 | 14 | 38 | 2 | 14 |
| Sausage, pepperoni & beef | 1 slice | 405 | 20 | 39 | 2 | 18 |
| Sausage & pepperoni | 1 slice | 348 | 15 | 38 | 2 | 16 |
| Vegetable garden fresh pizza | 1 slice | 287 | 9 | 40 | 3 | 12 |
| Works, the works pizza | 1 slice | 370 | 16 | 40 | 3 | 17 |
| Specialty pizzas | … | … | . | . | . | . |
| Alfredo, spinach | 1 slice | 303 | 12 | 37 | 2 | 13 |
| Alfredo, vegetable & chicken | 1 slice | 310 | 12 | 37 | 2 | 15 |
| Chicken and bacon BBQ | 1 slice | 370 | 14 | 44 | 2 | 17 |
| Hawaiian BBQ chicken | 1 slice | 375 | 14 | 46 | 2 | 17 |
| Thin crust pizza, large-14" | … | … | . | . | . | . |
| Cheese | 1 slice | 240 | 13 | 23 | 1 | 10 |
| Pepperoni | 1 slice | 295 | 18 | 23 | 2 | 12 |
| Sausage | 1 slice | 303 | 18 | 24 | 2 | 13 |
| Sausage, pepperoni & beef | 1 slice | 371 | 24 | 24 | 2 | 17 |
| Sausage & pepperoni | 1 slice | 298 | 18 | 23 | 1 | 13 |
| Vegetable garden fresh pizza | 1 slice | 228 | 11 | 24 | 2 | 9 |
| Works, the works pizza | 1 slice | 315 | 18 | 25 | 2 | 14 |

| FAST FOOD RESTAURANT: (See other Foods and Beverages listed separately) | Serving Size | Calories | Fat (g) | Carb (g) | Fiber (g) | Protein (g) |
|---|---|---|---|---|---|---|
| Specialty pizzas | ... | ... | . | . | . | . |
| Alfredo, spinach | 1 slice | 251 | 15 | 22 | 1 | 10 |
| Alfredo, vegetable & chicken | 1 slice | 276 | 15 | 22 | 1 | 14 |
| Chicken and bacon BBQ | 1 slice | 336 | 18 | 30 | 1 | 15 |
| Hawaiian BBQ chicken | 1 slice | 324 | 17 | 31 | 1 | 14 |
| Side items | ... | ... | . | . | . | . |
| BBQ dipping sauce | 1 svg | 48 | 0 | 10 | 0 | 0 |
| Bread sticks | 1 svg | 140 | 2 | 26 | 1 | 4 |
| Buffalo hot sauce | 1 svg | 25 | 1 | 3 | 0 | 0 |
| Cheese sauce | 1 svg | 60 | 5 | 0 | 0 | 4 |
| Cheese sticks | 1 svg | 180 | 8 | 20 | 1 | 8 |
| Chicken strips | 1 svg | 83 | 4 | 5 | Tr | 6 |
| Cinnapie | 1 svg | 114 | 6 | 14 | 0 | 1 |
| Garlic sauce | 1 svg | 235 | 26 | 0 | 0 | 0 |
| Honey mustard dipping sauce | 1 svg | 190 | 19 | 6 | 0 | 0 |
| Pizza sauce | 1 svg | 25 | 2 | 3 | 2 | 0 |
| Ranch dipping sauce | 1 svg | 140 | 14 | 2 | 0 | 1 |
| **Pizza Hut** | ... | ... | . | . | . | . |
| Bread stick | 1 | 130 | 4 | 20 | 1 | 3 |
| Bread stick sauce for dipping | 1 svg | 30 | 1 | 5 | 0 | 0 |
| Buffalo wings | 4 | 200 | 12 | 4 | 0 | 22 |
| Cavatini pasta | 1 svg | 485 | 14 | 66 | 9 | 21 |
| Cavatini pasta supreme | 1 svg | 565 | 19 | 73 | 10 | 24 |
| Cherry dessert pizza | 1 slice | 250 | 5 | 47 | 3 | 3 |
| Garlic bread | 1 slice | 150 | 8 | 16 | 1 | 3 |
| Ham and cheese sandwich | 1 | 555 | 21 | 57 | 4 | 33 |
| Hand tossed pizza | ... | ... | . | . | . | . |
| Beef | 1 slice | 260 | 9 | 16 | 2 | 16 |
| Cheese | 1 slice | 235 | 7 | 29 | 2 | 12 |
| Ham | 1 slice | 215 | 5 | 28 | 2 | 14 |
| Pepperoni | 1 slice | 238 | 8 | 28 | 2 | 13 |
| Sausage | 1 slice | 265 | 11 | 28 | 2 | 16 |
| Supreme | 1 slice | 284 | 12 | 29 | 3 | 13 |
| Pan pizza | ... | ... | . | . | . | . |
| Beef | 1 slice | 285 | 13 | 28 | 2 | 14 |
| Cheese | 1 slice | 260 | 11 | 28 | 2 | 12 |
| Ham | 1 slice | 240 | 9 | 28 | 2 | 11 |
| Pepperoni | 1 slice | 265 | 12 | 28 | 2 | 11 |
| Supreme | 1 slice | 310 | 15 | 28 | 3 | 15 |
| Veggie | 1 slice | 245 | 10 | 29 | 3 | 10 |
| Spaghetti with marina sauce | 1 svg | 490 | 6 | 91 | 8 | 18 |

| FAST FOOD RESTAURANT: (See other Foods and Beverages listed separately) | Serv- ing Size | Cal- ories | Fat (g) | Carb (g) | Fi- ber (g) | Pro- tein (g) |
|---|---|---|---|---|---|---|
| Spaghetti with meat sauce | 1 svg | 600 | 13 | 98 | 9 | 23 |
| Spaghetti with meatballs | 1 svg | 850 | 24 | 120 | 10 | 37 |
| Stuffed crust pizza | … | … | . | . | . | . |
|   Beef | 1 slice | 465 | 22 | 46 | 3 | 23 |
|   Cheese | 1 slice | 445 | 19 | 46 | 3 | 22 |
|   Ham | 1 slice | 404 | 22 | 45 | 3 | 24 |
|   Pepperoni | 1 slice | 440 | 19 | 45 | 3 | 21 |
|   Sausage | 1 slice | 480 | 23 | 46 | 3 | 22 |
| Supreme sandwich | 1 | 640 | 28 | 62 | 4 | 34 |
| Thin & crispy pizza | … | … | . | . | . | . |
|   Beef | 1 slice | 230 | 11 | 22 | 1 | 13 |
|   Cheese | 1 slice | 205 | 8 | 22 | 1 | 10 |
|   Pepperoni | 1 slice | 215 | 10 | 21 | 1 | 9 |
|   Sausage | 1 slice | 235 | 12 | 22 | 1 | 12 |
|   Supreme | 1 slice | 255 | 13 | 23 | 1 | 12 |
|   Veggie | 1 slice | 185 | 7 | 24 | 2 | 8 |
| **Subway** | … | … | . | . | . | . |
| Six Inch subs | … | … | . | . | . | . |
|   BLT on wheat | 1 | 325 | 10 | 44 | 3 | 14 |
|   BLT on white | 1 | 310 | 10 | 38 | 3 | 14 |
|   Classic Italian BMT wheat | 1 | 460 | 22 | 45 | 3 | 21 |
|   Classic Italian BMT white | 1 | 445 | 21 | 39 | 3 | 21 |
|   Cold cut trio on wheat | 1 | 380 | 13 | 46 | 3 | 20 |
|   Cold cut trio on white | 1 | 360 | 13 | 39 | 3 | 19 |
|   Ham on wheat | 1 | 300 | 5 | 45 | 3 | 19 |
|   Ham on white | 1 | 287 | 5 | 39 | 3 | 18 |
|   Meatball on wheat | 1 | 420 | 16 | 51 | 3 | 19 |
|   Meatball on white | 1 | 405 | 16 | 44 | 3 | 18 |
|   Pizza sub wheat | 1 | 465 | 22 | 48 | 3 | 19 |
|   Pizza sub white | 1 | 448 | 22 | 41 | 3 | 19 |
|   Roast beef on wheat | 1 | 305 | 5 | 45 | 3 | 20 |
|   Roast beef on white | 1 | 288 | 5 | 39 | 3 | 19 |
|   Roasted chicken breast, wheat | 1 | 348 | 6 | 47 | 3 | 27 |
|   Roasted chicken breast, white | 1 | 332 | 6 | 41 | 3 | 26 |
|   Spicy Italian wheat | 1 | 482 | 25 | 44 | 3 | 21 |
|   Spice Italian white | 1 | 465 | 24 | 38 | 3 | 20 |
|   Steak & cheese wheat | 1 | 395 | 10 | 47 | 3 | 30 |
|   Steak & cheese white | 1 | 383 | 10 | 41 | 3 | 29 |
|   Subway club wheat | 1 | 310 | 5 | 46 | 3 | 21 |
|   Subway club white | 1 | 295 | 5 | 40 | 3 | 21 |
|   Subway melt wheat | 1 | 382 | 12 | 46 | 3 | 23 |

| FAST FOOD RESTAURANT: (See other Foods and Beverages listed separately) | Serv-ing Size | Cal-ories | Fat (g) | Carb (g) | Fi-ber (g) | Pro-tein (g) |
|---|---|---|---|---|---|---|
| Subway melt white | 1 | 366 | 12 | 40 | 3 | 22 |
| Subway seafood & crab, wheat | 1 | 430 | 19 | 44 | 3 | 20 |
| Subway seafood & crab, white | 1 | 415 | 19 | 38 | 3 | 19 |
| Tuna on wheat | 1 | 542 | 32 | 44 | 3 | 19 |
| Tuna on white | 1 | 527 | 32 | 38 | 3 | 18 |
| Turkey breast & ham, wheat | 1 | 280 | 5 | 39 | 3 | 18 |
| Turkey breast & ham, white | 1 | 295 | 5 | 46 | 3 | 18 |
| Turkey on wheat | 1 | 289 | 4 | 46 | 3 | 18 |
| Turkey on white | 1 | 273 | 4 | 40 | 3 | 17 |
| Veggie delite wheat | 1 | 235 | 3 | 34 | 3 | 9 |
| Veggie delite white | 1 | 220 | 3 | 38 | 3 | 9 |
| Taco subs | … | … | . | . | . | . |
| Chicken taco sub wheat | 1 | 436 | 16 | 49 | 4 | 25 |
| Chicken taco sub white | 1 | 421 | 16 | 43 | 3 | 24 |
| Beverages | … | … | . | . | . | . |
| Berry lishus drink | small | 113 | 0 | 28 | 1 | 0 |
| Peach pizazz drink | small | 103 | 0 | 26 | 1 | 0 |
| Pineapple delight drink | small | 133 | 0 | 33 | 1 | 1 |
| Sunrise refresher drink | small | 119 | 0 | 29 | 1 | 1 |
| Cookies | … | … | . | . | . | . |
| Brazil nut & chocolate chip | 1 | 230 | 12 | 27 | 1 | 3 |
| Chocolate chip cookie | 1 | 210 | 10 | 29 | 1 | 2 |
| Chocolate chip, M&M cookie | 1 | 210 | 10 | 29 | 1 | 2 |
| Chocolate chunk cookie | 1 | 210 | 10 | 29 | 1 | 2 |
| Oatmeal raisin cookie | 1 | 205 | 8 | 29 | 1 | 3 |
| Peanut butter cookie | 1 | 220 | 12 | 26 | 1 | 3 |
| Sugar cookie | 1 | 230 | 12 | 28 | 0 | 2 |
| White chip macadamia nut | 1 | 235 | 12 | 28 | 0 | 2 |
| **Taco Bell** | … | … | . | . | . | . |
| Bacon cheeseburger | 1 | 565 | 30 | 43 | 4 | 29 |
| Bean burrito | 1 | 378 | 12 | 55 | 12 | 13 |
| Big beef meximelt | 1 | 300 | 16 | 21 | 2 | 16 |
| Big beef nachos supreme | 1 | 435 | 24 | 43 | 9 | 12 |
| Big beef supreme | 1 | 518 | 23 | 52 | 9 | 26 |
| Breakfast cheese quesadilla | 1 | 390 | 22 | 32 | 1 | 0 |
| Breakfast quesadilla with bacon | 1 | 465 | 28 | 33 | 1 | 1 |
| Breakfast quesadilla w/ sausage | 1 | 440 | 26 | 33 | 1 | 0 |
| Burrito supreme | 1 | 440 | 18 | 50 | 8 | 19 |
| Cheddar cheese | 1 svg | 30 | 2 | 0 | 0 | 2 |
| Cheese quesadilla | 1 | 370 | 20 | 32 | 1 | 16 |
| Chicken club | 1 | 540 | 31 | 43 | 4 | 22 |

| FAST FOOD RESTAURANT: (See other Foods and Beverages listed separately) | Serv- ing Size | Cal- ories | Fat (g) | Carb (g) | Fi- ber (g) | Pro- tein (g) |
|---|---|---|---|---|---|---|
| Chicken fajita | 1 | 460 | 21 | 49 | 3 | 18 |
| Chicken fajita supreme | 1 | 500 | 25 | 51 | 3 | 19 |
| Chicken quesadilla | 1 | 420 | 22 | 33 | 1 | 24 |
| Chili with cheese | 1 svg | 330 | 13 | 43 | 4 | 22 |
| Cinnamon twists | 1 svg | 140 | 6 | 19 | 0 | 1 |
| Country burrito | 1 | 270 | 14 | 26 | 1 | 1 |
| Double bacon & egg burrito | 1 | 480 | 27 | 39 | 2 | 2 |
| Double decker supreme | 1 | 390 | 18 | 39 | 8 | 16 |
| Double decker taco | 1 | 340 | 15 | 37 | 8 | 16 |
| Fiesta burrito | 1 | 280 | 16 | 25 | 1 | 1 |
| Grande burrito | 1 | 420 | 22 | 43 | 2 | 2 |
| Green sauce | 1 svg | 5 | 0 | 1 | 0 | 0 |
| Guacamole | 1 svg | 35 | 3 | 2 | 1 | 0 |
| Hot taco sauce | 1 svg | 1 | 0 | 0 | 0 | 0 |
| Kid's soft taco roll-up | 1 | 290 | 16 | 20 | 2 | 16 |
| Light chicken | 1 | 310 | 8 | 41 | 3 | 18 |
| Light chicken soft taco | 1 | 180 | 5 | 21 | 2 | 13 |
| Light chicken supreme | 1 | 430 | 13 | 52 | 3 | 25 |
| Light kid's chicken soft taco | 1 | 180 | 5 | 20 | 1 | 13 |
| Mexican pizza | 1 | 570 | 36 | 41 | 6 | 21 |
| Mexican rice | 1 svg | 190 | 10 | 20 | 0 | 6 |
| Mild taco sauce | 1 svg | 1 | 0 | 0 | 0 | 0 |
| Nacho cheese sauce | 1 svg | 120 | 10 | 5 | 0 | 2 |
| Nachos | 1 | 315 | 18 | 34 | 3 | 2 |
| Nachos belle grande | 1 | 740 | 39 | 83 | 17 | 16 |
| Pepper jack cheese | 1 svg | 25 | 2 | 1 | 0 | 0 |
| Picante sauce | 1 svg | 1 | 0 | 1 | 0 | 0 |
| Pinto & cheese | 1 | 195 | 8 | 18 | 10 | 9 |
| Red sauce | 1 svg | 10 | 0 | 2 | 0 | 0 |
| Salsa | 1 svg | 25 | 0 | 5 | 0 | 1 |
| Seven layer burrito | 1 | 540 | 24 | 65 | 14 | 16 |
| Soft taco | 1 | 210 | 10 | 20 | 2 | 12 |
| Soft taco, BLT | 1 | 340 | 23 | 22 | 2 | 11 |
| Soft taco, steak | 1 | 510 | 25 | 50 | 3 | 21 |
| Steak fajita | 1 | 465 | 21 | 49 | 3 | 18 |
| Taco, hard shell | 1 | 200 | 7 | 18 | 1 | 14 |
| Taco salad | 1 | 170 | 10 | 11 | 1 | 10 |
| Taco salad with salsa w/o shell | 1 | 420 | 21 | 29 | 13 | 26 |
| Taco supreme | 1 | 260 | 14 | 22 | 2 | 13 |
| Tostada | 1 | 305 | 14 | 31 | 11 | 11 |
| Veggie fajita | 1 | 420 | 19 | 51 | 3 | 11 |

| FAST FOOD RESTAURANT: (See other Foods and Beverages listed separately) | Serv-ing Size | Cal-ories | Fat (g) | Carb (g) | Fi-ber (g) | Pro-tein (g) |
|---|---|---|---|---|---|---|
| Veggie fajita supreme | 1 | 465 | 23 | 53 | 3 | 11 |
| **Wendy's** | ... | ... | . | . | . | . |
| Baked potato w/ bacon & cheese | 1 | 535 | 18 | 78 | 3 | 17 |
| Baked potato w/ broccoli, cheese | 1 | 470 | 14 | 80 | 3 | 9 |
| Baked potato with cheese | 1 | 570 | 23 | 78 | 3 | 14 |
| Baked potato w/ chili & cheese | 1 | 625 | 24 | 83 | 3 | 20 |
| Baked potato, sour cream, chive | 1 | 370 | 5 | 73 | 3 | 7 |
| Big bacon classic hamburger | 1 | 640 | 36 | 44 | 2 | 37 |
| Breaded chicken sandwich | 1 | 450 | 20 | 43 | 2 | 16 |
| Caesar salad | 1 | 110 | 6 | 6 | 2 | 9 |
| Cheeseburger kids' meal | 1 | 310 | 13 | 33 | 2 | 187 |
| Chicken Caesar pita | 1 | 485 | 19 | 48 | 2 | 30 |
| Chicken club sandwich | 1 | 520 | 25 | 44 | 3 | 30 |
| Chicken nuggets, 5 per svg | 1 svg | 190 | 13 | 9 | 2 | 9 |
| Chili (large) | 1 svg | 310 | 10 | 32 | 1 | 23 |
| Chili (small) | 1 svg | 210 | 7 | 21 | 1 | 15 |
| Chocolate chip cookie | 1 | 270 | 11 | 38 | 1 | 4 |
| Classic Greek pita | 1 | 440 | 20 | 50 | 1 | 16 |
| Classic hamburger, single | 1 | 360 | 16 | 45 | 1 | 24 |
| Classic hamburger w/ everything | 1 | 420 | 20 | 31 | 2 | 25 |
| Coleslaw | 1 svg | 45 | 3 | 5 | 1 | 0 |
| French fries (biggie) | 1 | 470 | 23 | 61 | 4 | 7 |
| French fries (small) | 1 | 270 | 13 | 35 | 2 | 4 |
| French fries (super) | 1 | 570 | 27 | 73 | 5 | 8 |
| Frosty (large) | 1 | 570 | 17 | 95 | 5 | 15 |
| Frosty (medium) | 1 | 460 | 13 | 76 | 4 | 12 |
| Frosty (small) | 1 | 340 | 10 | 57 | 3 | 9 |
| Garden ranch chicken pita | 1 | 480 | 18 | 51 | 2 | 27 |
| Garden veggie pita | 1 | 400 | 17 | 52 | 3 | 11 |
| Grilled chicken fillet, w/o bun | 1 | 100 | 3 | 0 | 0 | 19 |
| Grilled chicken salad | 1 | 190 | 8 | 10 | 2 | 22 |
| Grilled chicken sandwich | 1 | 290 | 7 | 35 | 2 | 24 |
| Hamburger kids' meal | 1 | 270 | 9 | 33 | 2 | 15 |
| Junior bacon cheeseburger | 1 | 445 | 25 | 33 | 2 | 22 |
| Junior cheeseburger | 1 | 320 | 13 | 34 | 2 | 18 |
| Junior cheeseburger deluxe | 1 | 360 | 17 | 36 | 2 | 18 |
| Junior hamburger | 1 | 270 | 9 | 34 | 2 | 15 |
| Kaiser bun | 1 | 190 | 3 | 36 | 2 | 6 |
| Sandwich bun | 1 | 160 | 3 | 29 | 2 | 5 |
| Spicy chicken sandwich | 1 | 415 | 15 | 43 | 3 | 28 |
| Strawberry banana dessert | 1 | 30 | 0 | 8 | 1 | Tr |

| FAST FOOD RESTAURANT: (See other Foods and Beverages listed separately) | Serving Size | Calories | Fat (g) | Carb (g) | Fiber (g) | Protein (g) |
|---|---|---|---|---|---|---|
| Taco salad | 1 | 375 | 19 | 28 | 1 | 26 |
| **White Castle** | .... | ... | . | . | . | . |
| Breakfast sandwich, regular | 1 | 335 | 25 | 17 | 1 | 14 |
| Cheeseburger | 1 | 235 | 14 | 11 | 1 | 7 |
| Cheeseburger with bacon | 1 | 200 | 13 | 12 | 1 | 10 |
| Cheeseburger, double | 1 | 285 | 18 | 12 | 1 | 14 |
| Cheesesticks, 5 per svg | 1 svg | 490 | 28 | 32 | 1 | 25 |
| Chicken rings, 6 per svg | 1 svg | 310 | 21 | 17 | 2 | 16 |
| Chicken ring sandwich | 1 | 170 | 7 | 15 | 2 | 5 |
| Chocolate shake | 14 oz | 220 | 7 | 32 | 1 | 8 |
| Fish sandwich | 1 | 160 | 6 | 18 | 1 | 8 |
| French fries, small | 1 | 115 | 6 | 15 | 1 | 1 |
| Hamburger | 1 | 135 | 7 | 11 | 1 | 6 |
| Hamburger, double | 1 | 235 | 14 | 16 | 1 | 11 |
| Onion rings, 8 per svg | 1 svg | 455 | 25 | 45 | 1 | 12 |
| Vanilla shake | 14 oz | 228 | 7 | 35 | 0 | 8 |

# EASY LIFETIME
# DIET & EXERCISE GUIDE

It is possible to take total control of your weight. The facts, tips, and ideas in this guide provide the "need to know" essentials of calories, exercise, and weight management. This guide along with the calorie counter gives the power and the knowledge for permanent solutions to weight management, while promoting good overall health.

This plan is safe, effective, easy to follow, and fits into any lifestyle. Learn the secrets to weight management, and simple exercise routines that lead to a lifetime of health, well being, and total success in weight control.

Fad diets, crash diets, and starvation diets are not recommended. Any temporary weight loss on a crash diet, will return quickly once normal eating habits are resumed. There are also potential adverse health effects from any type of quick weight loss diet, and data shows that starvation diets also lead to a slower metabolism.

For total lifetime weight management, it is better to have a diet plan that is fairly easy to maintain on a permanent basis; one that hardly feels like a diet at all.

This diet plan is very simple: First choose your ideal body weight. You may know exactly what is right for you, or you can refer to the "Ideal Body Weight" chart. You then calculate the number of daily calories needed to achieve that weight. (Calculations discussed later). You can eat satisfying and well-balanced variety of foods, including all your favorite foods, while making better food choices by counting calories. Read over the Healthy Diet Basics, and the Easy Weight Loss Secrets. If you want to achieve optimal health, you should add a simple exercise routine to your day. Exercise also helps speed up weight loss, and makes lifetime weight management much easier.

When trying to lose weight, several factors come into play that affect the speed of weight loss. This includes:

- How many pounds you are above your ideal weight. Generally, the more you weigh, the faster you will lose weight. Losing and keeping off the last 10 pounds is usually the most difficult. Losing 5 to 7 pounds per month is a healthy goal.
- Your commitment to counting and cutting calories; and your commitment to get active with exercise.
- Your metabolism. As you age, metabolism naturally slows down. Exercise speeds up the metabolism. Heredity is also a factor; some people have a faster metabolism than others.

## **Healthy Diet Basics**

The following is a list of important facts, and healthy tips to keep in mind for smart weight management. These tips will help in achieving and maintaining your ideal weight.

Drink 6 to 8 glasses of water every day. Water helps to cleanse and purify the body, and improves overall health.

Take a multi-vitamin and mineral supplement every day. This helps to assure that you are obtaining all the essential nutrients your body needs.

Eat a variety of foods every day from all of the food groups. Variety and balance in the food groups helps to assure proper nutrition and good health. All types of foods contain varying amounts of vitamins, minerals, and nutrients. The food groups are:

- Bread, grains, oats, wheat, cereal, rice, and pasta.
  (Good source of carbs and fiber, some protein).

- Fruits and vegetables.
  (Fruits and vegetables contain many

nutrients, fiber, and antioxidants).

- Dairy products including milk, and cheese.
  (High in protein and carbs, some are high in fat).

- Meat products including beef, pork, chicken, fish, and eggs.
  (High in protein, some are high in fat).

- Fats, oils, and sweets. Minimize intake of this food group.
  (Very high in fat and/or sugar).

The USDA recommendations for variety and balance in daily caloric intake follows:

- 50% to 60% from carbohydrates
- 12% to 20% from proteins
- Less than 30% from fats

For example, in an 1800 calorie diet, for a 120 pound adult, the USDA recommends the following daily intake for optimal nutritional health:

Carbohydrates: 250 grams
                (about 55% of total caloric intake)

Protein:  54 grams
                (about 16% of total caloric intake)

Fat:  Less than 58 grams
                (less than 30% of total caloric intake)

Fiber: 23 grams or more. Fiber is found in carbohydrates and supplies multiple health benefits. Fiber is especially good for the heart and colon. Some studies indicate that an increase in fiber with the proper balance of protein increases the metabolism naturally, resulting in faster weight loss, and easier weight management.

Carbohydrates can be classified as simple, such as sugar, or complex. The complex carbohydrates are healthy and contain many nutrients. Carbohydrates also include fiber. Foods high in complex carbs, such as bread and rice contain many vitamins and minerals. Carbs also contain starch and sugar. Sugar is the so-called "bad carb"; high in calories with little nutritional value. You can usually identify a bad carb because it is sweet.

Some diets promote higher intake of protein, with lower intake of carbohydrates. This does promote faster weight loss in many people, however, nutrition experts agree that a well balanced diet with higher intake of carbohydrates, less protein, and less fat is safer and healthier. A minor increase in protein intake, with a minor decrease in carbohydrate intake is a better option if considering a high protein/low carb diet. The extremes of almost all protein and fat, with almost no carbohydrate intake can have serious health consequences. Many high protein foods are also high in fat and cholesterol, and some are high in sodium (processed meats). Health problems noted in high protein, high fat, low carb diets include: kidney failure, increased risk of heart disease due to increased cholesterol levels, and increased risk of cancer.

# All About Calories & Weight

**Simply put, if you eat fewer calories, you will lose weight.** There are 3500 calories in one pound. For every 3500 calories you cut out of your diet, you will lose one pound of body weight. Calories provide energy. You need calories and the energy derived from calories to live. However, if you consume more calories than your body needs, the result is weight gain. For the safest, healthiest weight loss, you need to maintain the proper caloric intake, balance your food groups, and increase your physical activity level. This leads to good health, good nutrition, and easy to maintain, long lasting results.

You can choose your perfect weight for yourself, or refer to the ideal body weight chart. Then you just determine the number of calories you need per day to achieve that weight. For example: Let's say your ideal weight is 120 pounds, and you have a moderately active lifestyle. You need approximately 1800 calories per day. (See the lifestyle activity levels and factors). 1800 calories per day is a satisfying amount of food in most people's opinion. 1800 calories per day leaves plenty of room for good variety, balance, and nutrition. You just need to learn to make smart food choices, and counting calories is the best way.

Read over the calorie counter. Get to know which foods are naturally lower in calories. Reducing your caloric intake, and managing your weight is so much easier once you learn which types of foods are high in calories, and which types of foods are low in calories.

Calorie counting gets easier over time, and after a while it is like second nature. After a few months of using a calorie counter, most people have memorized the approximate calorie counts of favorite foods. While it is true every calorie counts in weight management, it is also true that every bit of activity also counts. It is almost impossible to measure exactly how many calories you burn in a day; you would have to measure calorie expenditure every time you stand up, even every time you move. It is, however, easy to figure approximately how many calories you need, and how many you burn per day with the simple formulas in this book. So, you do not need to spend lots of time counting every calorie. Instead, try rounding and averaging calories to save time, but don't cheat yourself by neglecting to count the majority of your calories.

After some practice counting calories, you won't even need to write down the daily calorie counts. Many experienced calorie counting people are able to keep a daily running total in the back of their mind.

## How many calories do you need per day?

There are complicated formulas and expensive tests to determine your caloric requirements based on basal metabolism. A very simple rule of thumb is to choose your ideal weight and multiply by 15 to determine your daily caloric requirements. This formula is correct for moderately active, healthy adults over age 18. The activity levels and factors are discussed in the next section.

If you are extremely active, your caloric requirements will be higher. If you are sedentary, your caloric requirements will be lower.

Caloric requirements decrease with age as the metabolism slows down. Every 5-10 years, you will likely notice a few pounds creeping on despite your best efforts. You will need to consume slightly less calories and/or exercise a little more to stay at the same weight. Note: Caloric requirements can be significantly increased during any illness. Caloric requirements can be reduced in cases of hypothyroidism.

# Formula for Calculating Daily Calories Needed:

Multiply your ideal body weight by your activity factor to determine daily caloric requirements.

**Example:** A moderately active adult who wants to weigh 120 pounds, needs 1800 calories per day.

$$120 \times 15 = 1800$$

# Lifestyle Activity Levels & Factors

**Sedentary Lifestyle   (Factor = 12)**
  Sitting most of the day, no formal exercise program.

**Moderately Active Lifestyle   (Factor = 15)**
  Performs regular moderately strenuous exercise
  program at least 3 times per week for at least 20

minutes per session. Good amount of walking and activity in normal daily routine.

## Vigorously Active Lifestyle   (Factor = 18)

Extremely active.  Performs regular strenuous exercise at least 5 times per week for at least 30 minutes per session.  Exercise program includes running or jogging at fast pace, high impact aerobic type exercise, or equally strenuous exercise. Daily routine and/or job include lots of physical activity.

**If you fall somewhere in the middle, your activity factor will fall somewhere in the middle of these activity factors.**

Calorie expenditure describes the process of the body utilizing or burning calories for energy.  Different activities burn calories at different levels.  You can measure your overall lifestyle activity level and the factors by using this chart.  You can then make adjustments to your activity level, and add exercises that help burn calories faster.

Tip:  Every time you perform a physical activity or exercise, you are burning more calories than if you are sitting.  So a key to losing weight faster, is to GET ACTIVE!  Take the stairs whenever possible, take a walk after eating, find an exercise or activity you enjoy, and add it to your daily routine.  Adding a simple exercise like walking, biking, or swimming to your daily routine, for 20 minutes per day, 3 to 5 days per week will help to speed up weight loss, increase muscle tone, and increase your energy level.

Note: As you age your metabolism naturally slows down. Even expert lifelong diet and exercise enthusiasts report that around age 30 to 40 they have to eat a little less or exercise a little more to maintain the same weight; and they report that about every 5 to 10 years as the metabolism slows down, they need to adjust their diet and exercise plan slightly in order to maintain the same weight.

## Which exercises burn more calories?

Simply, the more strenuous the exercise, the more calories you burn. You can also gauge how vigorous the exercise is by checking your heart rate. (This is discussed later.)

Weight training/weightlifting is a little different than other exercises. You may or may not increase you heart rate as much as with other exercises, but you are still doing yourself a world of good. Weight training is very effective at toning muscles and increasing lean muscle mass. This means you will have less fat and more muscle on your body. Muscle also weighs more than fat, so you will need more calories per day to maintain your weight. You can also achieve your ideal physique by adjusting the amount of weights you train with, and the number of repetitions you perform. You can choose to be anywhere from lean and well-toned to very muscular. To achieve that, women can use light weights and more repetitions. Men can use heavier weights with less repetitions.

An exercise is classified as aerobic if you can achieve and maintain your maximum heart rate range for at least 20 minutes, and preferably 30 minutes. Aerobic exercise provides a multitude of health benefits:
- Increased energy levels
- Faster weight loss
- Improved overall health
- Lower blood pressure and lower resting heart rate (This is a long-term beneficial aspect of aerobic exercise).

Before beginning an exercise, check your normal resting heart rate. The normal for an adult is 60 to 100 beats per minute, with 80 being the average normal value. Count the heartbeat for 15 seconds and multiply by 4 to calculate beats per minute. Then check your heart rate periodically while performing an exercise, to be sure you are maintaining the aerobic level.

## Using heart rate to calculate aerobic exercise level:

**Your target heart rate while exercising is calculated as follows:**

**220 (minus your age) x ( 75%)**

Example: for a 35-year-old:
220 – 35 = 185  x  75%  = 139

In this example, the 35-year-old can gauge the exercise activity level by the heart rate increase from a resting heart rate of 80 to the aerobic exercise heart rate of 139. The heart rate should be checked periodically to gauge the aerobic level.

Note: If your heart rate is much higher than calculated in the formula, you should stop exercising, and consult your physician before restarting aerobic exercise. Also, any illness including a fever can increase heart rate, so the heart rates given here are for normal healthy adults only. Always check with your doctor before beginning any exercise program.

Calorie expenditure increases with more strenuous exercise and activity. This chart reveals some common activities and the number of calories burned per hour during these activities.

# Calorie expenditure chart*

| Activity/Exercise | *Calories burned per hour | |
| --- | :---: | :---: |
| | **Female** | **Male** |
| Sitting quietly | **60** | **80** |
| Standing still | **75** | **100** |
| Light activity/exercise<br>  Cleaning the house<br>  Walking slowly/strolling<br>  Playing golf<br>  Light weight training/weightlifting | **210** | **250** |
| Moderate activity/exercise<br>  Bicycling at 6 mph<br>  Fast power walking at 3.5 mph<br>  Swimming at a moderate pace<br>  Low/Moderate impact aerobics<br>  Dancing at moderate pace<br>  Moderate weight training/weightlifting<br>  Playing basketball or tennis | **330** | **410** |
| Strenuous activity/exercise<br>  High impact aerobics<br>  Swimming very fast<br>  Jogging/running at 8 mph or faster<br>  Jumping rope very fast<br>  Stair stepping<br>  Cross country skiing | **620** | **800** |

*Calories burned per hour in this example are approximate values for a normal healthy adult female weighing 130 pounds, or a normal, healthy adult male weighing 165 pounds.

# Activity / Exercise Tips

**Choose an activity you enjoy, and perform it regularly for at least 20 minutes per day, at least three days per week.** This will promote faster weight loss, easier weight management, improved overall health, and improved sense of well being.

This exercise can be as simple as walking. You can walk outside, or use a treadmill, or simulate a walk inside while watching your favorite television program, or catching up on the news. You should walk at a fast pace, but one that is comfortable to you. Don't walk so fast that you get short of breath. Your stamina and endurance will increase the longer you continue. If you are walking inside, be sure to really lift your feet off the floor. As you walk, be sure to swing your arms back and forth.

Other simple methods include bicycling outdoors or on an indoor stationary bike. Also try performing aerobics with an exercise video, kickboxing video, or dance video, in endless varieties of styles and speeds. Choose light aerobics first and work your way up to high impact aerobics when that feels comfortable.

If you want to tone up your muscles faster, and burn lots of extra calories, you can hold weights in your hands while you exercise. You can also try strapping weights on your wrists and ankles while you are exercising, while working around the house, taking a walk, or riding a stationary bike. Start with low weights like one pound weights for the arms and two or three pound weights for the ankles. Lifting or swinging the arms up over the head gets the heart rate up much faster and burns more calories. You can increase these weights as you get used to them. **This is an easy, effective and inexpensive way to tone muscles.**

Once you have mastered one exercise, you can step up to a higher activity level exercise. Read over the list to see which ones burn more calories, and find one you truly enjoy. Once you have achieved your ideal weight, continue the exercise routine, or even step up a level, to maintain optimal good health and the ideal weight.

## Easy Weight Loss Secrets

**Try these tips for fast and easy weight loss. Step on the scale a week later, or a month later and be amazed at the results. Be sure to also follow the Healthy Diet Basics outlined earlier.**

- Many of your favorite foods come in low calorie, light, sugar free, low fat, and fat free versions that taste great. Try several until you find some you like. The result of switching to the low calorie versions of foods and drinks is fast and easy weight loss. Try switching for ¼ or ½ of the foods and beverages you consume, and be amazed at the results.

- Do splurge occasionally and do include your favorite foods in your lifetime weight management plan. Everyone wants to enjoy special foods and drinks for holidays, special occasions, eating out with friends, and just because it's good to treat yourself.

- Remember that almost everything is good for you IN MODERATION! Even a chocolate bar has some health benefits. Enjoy what you love in moderation, and don't let excess destroy your diet.

- After the special occasions, you can easily get right back into the pattern of healthy eating. Many successful dieters occasionally skip the meat dish or the side dish, and instead enjoy the dessert or other favorites. This is a guilt-free option that won't be hard to work off.

- By switching to the sugar free or calorie-free version of most of your beverages, you can cut your daily caloric intake considerably; even up to 800 calories per day, with very little effort.

- When you choose foods in the low calorie, light, sugar free, low fat, or fat free versions, you save anywhere from 10% to 90% of the calories for that dish. For example, a rice dish made with 1 tablespoon of regular butter has 250 calories. If you use fat free margarine instead of regular butter, the total calories are about 150, saving you 100 calories. A salad with 2 tablespoons of fat free dressing instead of regular dressing saves you about 120 calories.

- Prepare your food without adding cooking oil that has 120 calories per tablespoon. Try baking, broiling, or grilling with a non-stick cooking spray that has zero calories.

- With sugar free fruit flavored beverages like *Crystal Light* or *Kool Aid*, you can save about 100 calories per cup over regular fruit flavored beverages. These come in many varieties and are excellent thirst quenchers. With soft drinks, you can reduce the calories from about 150 to zero by switching to a diet version of the soda.

- For between meal snacks, try anything low calorie, and low fat. Some examples are sugar free gum and candy, vegetables with fat free dip, carrot sticks, pretzels, crackers, and any diet beverage. With just a small snack you will easily be able to curb your cravings for an hour or two until your next meal.

- **Choose foods that are low in fat, salt, and sugar. These foods are naturally lower in calories and promote weight loss.** High fat diets have multiple detrimental effects to your health in addition to weight gain. Also avoid high sodium foods to avoid water retention weight gain. Sodium or salt intake should be minimized. High sodium diets can detrimentally affect your entire cardiovascular system, including your heart, and can detrimentally increase your blood pressure. Most processed foods and restaurant foods are high in sodium already, so there is no need to add salt. Try adding just a bit of pepper instead. When eating at home, try to switch to a salt-free substitute, or, if this is too bland, then try to use a mixture of ½ salt, and ½ salt substitute. This substitute of ½ each is healthier, lowers your salt intake, and also tastes great! Add a dash of pepper on top or a dash of cayenne powder to spice it up. **Also, when shopping, look at generic store brands which are almost always lower in calories, salt/sodium, and fat than name-brand foods, and many of these taste great.**

- Many successful dieters take a multi-vitamin/mineral supplement every day including a calcium supplement. (Many vitamins do not supply the recommended daily amount of calcium.) They also take herbal supplements including a daily fruit and vegetable tablet, and a daily apple cider vinegar plus green tea supplement. These herbal supplements provide a variety of health benefits, and some claim they can help promote weight loss. Also, if you are unable to get all the fruits and vegetables in your diet every day, this will be a good replacement with near zero calories. Take these with meals and be sure to drink 6-8 glasses of water daily.

- **Add a little physical activity at least three to five days per week.** Read the fitness guide which includes calorie expenditure charts as related to exercise. To begin, choose a simple and pleasant exercise such as walking, swimming, or riding a bicycle. Just 20 minutes per day, a few days per week, can dramatically accelerate your weight loss, increase energy levels, and improve your overall sense of well being. Your brain releases endorphins when you exercise. Endorphins are chemicals that make you feel good, and the feeling can last for many hours after you finish exercising. Many people who exercise regularly say they feel energized all day long.

Please Note: As with any weight management plan, results may vary for each individual. You should always consult your physician before beginning any new diet or exercise plan; and especially if you have current health problems, or you are pregnant or nursing. This diet plan is offered only as information, for use in maintaining and promoting good health. In the event that the information presented in this diet plan is used without a physician's approval, the individual using the plan accepts all responsibility. This plan is only intended for healthy adults over age 18. Always consult your physician first.

# Ideal Body Weight Chart

The following chart is to help calculate ideal body weight for adults. The data is compiled from various health journals. There is a wide range of what is considered to be the "ideal" body weight. This chart lists weights for a medium frame, with one to two pounds of clothing on. Heights listed are without shoes. It is best to weigh yourself in the morning, before eating or drinking anything. This is the best way to track the trend of your weight loss. Weight can fluctuate throughout the day, especially after eating a meal. Use this chart only as an estimated guide to your ideal weight.

## FEMALE:

| Height (Feet' Inches") | Ideal Body Weight (in Pounds) |
|---|---|
| 5'0" | 100 – 110 |
| 5'1" | 102 – 112 |
| 5'2" | 105 – 118 |
| 5'3" | 108 – 122 |
| 5'4" | 110 – 125 |
| 5"5" | 114 – 130 |
| 5'6" | 116 – 136 |
| 5'7" | 120 – 140 |
| 5'8" | 125 – 145 |
| 5'10" | 130 – 155 |

## MALE:

| Height (Feet' Inches") | Ideal Body Weight (in Pounds) |
|---|---|
| 5'4" | 125 – 140 |
| 5'6" | 135 – 155 |
| 5'8" | 145 – 165 |
| 5'10" | 160 – 175 |
| 6'0" | 170 – 185 |
| 6'2" | 180 – 195 |

*Let's face it, we all want to be lean and toned while not having to put in extraordinary effort. This book gives you all the secrets to safe, easy, effective, and permanent results in managing your weight. You can enjoy a lifetime of optimal health at your perfect weight. Inside, find the power and the knowledge to control your weight forever. No fad diets or extreme maneuvers are going to work for long. We all need permanent and easy-to-follow solutions to stay physically fit.*

*First, you need a fast & easy to use calorie & nutrient counter to help you make smart food choices. Whether you are a pro, or a novice at counting calories, you will find this book contains all the data you need for fast, easy, accurate food counts. Experts agree calories count first in weight management. The EASY Lifetime Diet & Exercise Guide is included to help you lose weight faster, and shape and tone your body, while achieving optimal health. Included is information about understanding calories, understanding calorie expenditure, lifestyle activity factors, and simple tips for achieving your goals. This book contains the essential tools for easy lifetime weight management.*

*Inside find all the foods you love to eat. All the most popular and most common foods, fast food restaurants, brand names, beverages, and alcohol. About 3,500 listings included. Available in print edition or ebook for download to your favorite device.*

Made in the USA
Middletown, DE
23 June 2018